On a Desperate Journey

Get off the diet treadmill!

Written by Mia T. Sutherland
Copyright 2007

Order this book online at www.trafford.com/07-0097
or email orders@trafford.com

Most Trafford titles are also available at major online book retailers.

Note for Librarians: A cataloguing record for this book is available from Library
and Archives Canada at www.collectionscanada.ca/amicus/index-e.html

Printed in Victoria, BC, Canada.

ISBN: 978-1-4251-1725-2

*We at Trafford believe that it is the responsibility of us all, as both individuals
and corporations, to make choices that are environmentally and socially sound.
You, in turn, are supporting this responsible conduct each time you purchase a
Trafford book, or make use of our publishing services. To find out how you are
helping, please visit www.trafford.com/responsiblepublishing.html*

*Our mission is to efficiently provide the world's finest, most comprehensive
book publishing service, enabling every author to experience success.
To find out how to publish your book, your way, and have it available
worldwide, visit us online at www.trafford.com/10510*

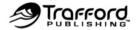

www.trafford.com

North America & international
toll-free: 1 888 232 4444 (USA & Canada)
phone: 250 383 6864 ♦ fax: 250 383 6804
email: info@trafford.com

The United Kingdom & Europe
phone: +44 (0)1865 722 113 ♦ local rate: 0845 230 9601
facsimile: +44 (0)1865 722 868 ♦ email: info.uk@trafford.com

10 9 8 7 6 5 4 3

This book is dedicated to my mom for never saying the word diet when I was growing up. For always being concerned about nutrition and family values. For being proud of her job as a mother and a wife. For never making weight an issue and for loving who she was, the way she was.

ACKNOWLEDGEMENTS

Without the support, insight and courage of many people I would not have had the opportunity to put these ideas on paper. I would like to start by thanking the 160 women and girls that participated in this project. Your time, your courage, and your energy were inspirational and enlightening to say the least. The counselors and teachers who helped organize the student panel discussions and the Superintendent of School District 71, thank you—without your participation many of the issues surrounding this dilemma would not have been addressed.

Nancy Newsom and Kathy Jerritt, thank you for the many hours spent editing this project. I didn't realize how lazy my grammar had become. My friends and family for believing in this project and encouraging me to continue when I expressed concern about what I had gotten myself into. My brother Boomer Jerritt of Strathcona Photography, for doing an amazing job of the cover. A special thank you to Tracy Severin and Nancy Newsom for teaching me, early in my career, that weight loss can be achieved through hard work, determination and dignity and for allowing me to come along on the journey. Tracy, wherever you are, I hope you see this acknowledgement.

I would like to thank my son for always asking how the book was going and for giving me much needed hugs when I was locked away in my office typing for hours on end. Lastly, thank you to my husband for encouraging me to not "work" for a while. Without that encouragement, I would not have had the opportunity to take on such an overwhelming project.

TABLE OF CONTENTS

FOREWORD

Let me start by saying that I am not a counselor, a therapist, a psychologist or a psychiatrist. I'm not a nutritionist or a dietician. I've never suffered from an eating disorder or from weight issues. I don't have a degree and I'm not a writer. I am simply someone with immense empathy and curiosity. I am also someone who worked in an industry for 20 years that gave people permission to obsess about their bodies. When I retired from the fitness industry a nagging curiosity got the best of me and I began to read and to research, to ask questions and to talk to people about their experiences with food and with weight and with body image. The common threads and frustrating ironies kept me nibbling at the edge of this complex, exasperating and desperate epidemic. This book is a journey of voices brought together in order to bring the reader insight and more importantly, hope. It is not a book about eating disorders and it is not another diet book. It is a *how-to* book and it is a *why* book. Perhaps if we ask enough questions, eventually we will ask the right ones and from these questions will come answers. What the answer is for one reader may be entirely different for another reader. As long as the questions get answered or the reader finds hope, this book has been a success and my goal has been achieved.

This book comes from years of working with women in fitness. When we talk about women and exercise the sub-title usually reads, "I am starting an exercise program because I am unhappy with the way I look" not, "I am starting an exercise program because I want to have more energy when I play with my child", or "I want to lower my blood pressure", or "I want to alleviate stress". I found it shocking that extremely intelligent women with Masters degrees and PhDs, Doctors, entrepreneurs, nurses, professional athletes and all walks of life suffer from the same issues with food, weight, low self-esteem and distorted body image. Intelligent, motivated, focused, determined women who completely lose their ability to rationalize their physical self-perception, relative to an unrealistic bar set by the media, by our friends, by our families and by ourselves. The unrealistic bar is different for each woman. It may be a movie star, a model, the woman next door, an athlete, your sister, or your mother.

The irony is two-fold. The women and girls we are trying to emulate have a professional team that spend hours doing hair and makeup as well as organizing clothing that accentuates their clients strengths, such as long legs, and hides their perceived weaknesses, such as wide hips. These women are successful based on their external appearance not their internal composition. I watched an interview with one of America's premiere models and she complained once the magazines had finished stretching out her figure and airbrushing away imperfections, she would cringe at the thought of going on a date because she didn't' look like the magazine ads. We put tremendous pressure on ourselves to achieve an image that isn't real.

Perhaps the greater irony is the reality that most of the women we are aspiring to look like, want to look like someone else. Larger breasts, longer legs, blonder hair, curly hair, straight hair, thinner, curvier, taller, shorter and so on and so on. When we begin to appreciate and to love ourselves for who we are and what we have, we will have begun the journey home to a happier, more peaceful place.

One of the women interviewed for this book said to me the saddest thing about turning 40 was that she had spent the last 20 years trying to become someone and something other than who she was. She had struggled with food and body-image on a daily/hourly basis. She had two beautiful children, a husband and a successful career but the one thing that consumed her time was her daily struggle with her relationship with food, body-image and weight. The irony was, she had a body that was the envy of most women who came in contact with her.

I hope this book makes women realize that they are not alone. There are solutions. We can laugh at ourselves and this insanity and just because we do insane things, doesn't mean we are insane. This struggle with this demon does not define who we are and on this desperate journey, there is hope.

1
WHY?

Sticks and stones can break my bones but words can never hurt me. Fat cow. I hate you. You're ugly. Stupid. You're fat. Get a life. I don't love you anymore. Fat ass. She is my new best friend. She is prettier. Those pants make you look like a hippo. You have a face like a dog. You're getting chubby. You stink. Get over it. Move on. Do something with your hair. You need to lose weight, lots of weight. What's wrong with your face?

Words have the power to break a person's spirit. They have the ability to destroy self-esteem, butcher self-confidence and distort personal perceptions. It was amazing how many women I spoke with who could pinpoint the exact moment in time—20, 30, 40 years ago when little Suzie said such and such, and that planted the seed. The seed, when watered and fertilized with the wrong messages, the wrong words and the wrong perceptions, would grow to dictate and to control and to destroy the lives of otherwise healthy women.

Where do our beliefs come from? We are not born wondering why our legs are short and chubby or why we have a Buddha belly or why it's okay to lay around naked. These, like so many facets of our lives, are learned traits and they are learned from external environments and messages. Messages we receive from our parents and siblings. Messages we receive from our friends. Messages that are pounded into our brains through the media. Messages through music and movies and commercials. Messages from boys and from men, from brothers and from husbands. If we don't have the confidence or the tools to understand those messages are a reflection of the person or the place they are coming from, we begin to believe what is said. The media is hoping that if you see enough commercials about anti-wrinkle cream, you will begin to think you need the cream. If you see enough ads about covering up the grey, you'll think you need to dye your hair. If your husband tells you enough times that you are fat and useless, eventually you begin to believe that you are. It is critical that we learn to control our minds in order to sort through the truth—not let our minds control us. We need to start taking each and every experience in life and use it as a lesson to learn from, instead of allowing ourselves to become a victim of it. This chapter is dedicated to all the women reading this book that can remember the exact moment in time when the journey of self-loathing began.

"I remember my mom used to always say to me, 'Butterflies come in pretty colors and elephants only come in grey.' I knew she meant I was grey." **Interview client #14**

"When I was 18 or 19, I had someone that was close to me at the time tell me that I had an odd-shaped body. In my mind,

I half defended myself and half believed him.”
Interview client #35

“I remember when I was 12 or 13, the style was to wear bell
bottom jeans with a body suit. I was so proud when I got my
very first pair of bell bottoms. I put them on and came down-
stairs to show my mom. She said, ‘Well your abs need work but
other than that it’s not too bad.’ I never wore the outfit.”
Interview client #46

“I remember a boyfriend telling me that having my hair short
in the back made my ass look big.”
Interview client #27

“My mother was always saying, ‘If only you could lose weight, I
could buy you clothes that fit’.”   **Interview client #11**

“I do remember several times in the past 20 years the positive
comments that I have received on the way that I look and how
it has affected the way I feel about my body.”
Interview client #13

“When I was younger my husband used to question everything
I was eating and how much of everything I was eating. I be-
came very self-conscious about eating around him.”
Interview client #22

“My mom yo-yo dieted all of her life and my life. She shared
her emotional eating with us and my dad used to make negative remarks like, ‘Why eat that pie—just give it to your thighs
because it’s going there anyway’.” **Interview client #68**

“My friends ask why I’m so fat.”   **Student**

Do as I say not as I do.

I watched a talk show not long ago and the guest was a mother and her 120 pound three-year-old son. When the woman was asked why her child was so overweight, she responded by saying she had taken the child to every doctor she could think of and no one could find anything wrong with him. When asked what the child ate, she commented that it wasn't anything out of the ordinary. Three eggs, bacon, sausage and toast for breakfast, mid-morning snacks, pre-lunch snacks, pasta or pizza or sandwiches for lunch, mid-afternoon snacks, pre-dinner snacks and so on. Not only was his diet absurd but the amount of food at each sitting was enormous. When I listened to her, it was obvious where the problem was coming from. He was three, and only knew what he was taught. The child was eventually removed from the mother's care and was placed in foster care where he lost 70 pounds.

The old saying, *Do as I say not as I do*, should be kept on a post-it-note on the bathroom mirror. If you tell your daughter to love her body and treat it with respect but you use inappropriate sexual behavior to get a date, she will get mixed messages. If you tell your daughter it is okay to be heavier than her best friend but you constantly compare yourself to your neighbor, she will get the message. If you tell your daughter not to eat unconsciously but you snack on junk food while driving to and from soccer practice, she will get the picture. If you can't live what you are preaching, then it is time for you to deal with your food issues before you show your daughter the path to a long, painful road.

"My mom will lie on the bed and say that she likes the way her hip bones stick out when she is lying down."
Grade 6 student

"My mom always stands in her underwear and bra in front of the mirror and asks me if I think she looks fat. I hate it when she asks me because she's not but I know she doesn't believe me." **Grade 5 student**

What we say and how we conduct ourselves around the issue of food and weight will likely have a direct correlation on how our daughters feel and conduct themselves around food. Establishing a fine line between educating, guiding, nurturing and supporting our daughters throughout their food formative years versus nagging, chastising, forcing food, hiding food and negative self-talk, becomes as individual between you and your daughter as the relationship between you and food.

"When I was very young, I remember that what I looked like was a constant focus. Unfortunately I remember most of this pressure from my mother, which you can imagine has caused many strained times in our relationship. It was never a focus for my dad, as I always felt that I could do no wrong in his eyes. I can't say the same for my mom, and I still get very bitter when I think of things that she said, did, insinuated, teased, when I was growing up. I clearly remember this starting at Christmas when I was eight." **Interview client #13**

Loving food is easier than loving yourself.

We connect physical nourishment (the act of eating) with emotional nourishment (making us feel something). We refer to our loved ones by food nurturing names such as pumpkin, peanut, honey, sweetie, pea, sugar, carrot top. They all have warm, comforting meanings and they make us feel happy emotionally, just like eating makes us feel happy physically. Recognizing whether we are eating to feel satisfied because we are hungry or we are eating so we don't have to feel an emotion that makes us uncomfortable, such as loneliness, boredom, stress, fear, fatigue or anxiety, is essential to a healthy food relationship.

Hand-to-mouth eating has the potential to be one of our most disastrous food habits. That is the act of eating when you are not hungry and are simply unconsciously putting food in your mouth without enjoying it or tasting it. Typical late night eating. Author Susie Orbach refers to it as *stomach hungry* and *mouth hungry*. Being able to recognize the difference is like admitting you have a problem. "Hello, my name is Martha and I have a hand-to-mouth disorder!" Many times it isn't necessarily what you are eating that is the problem but why, when and how much. So many people think if they would just start eating low fat, their weight problems will go away.

Fat is an essential nutrient, but not in the quantity that it is being consumed. Women are so afraid of fat, of being fat, of eating fat, of looking fat, of getting fat, of seeing fat, of touching fat. People struggling with weight issues or judging people with weight issues need to realize that being fat does not necessarily mean being unhealthy. Some of us are genetically predisposed to be fatter than our friends, neighbors, siblings. Some people, contrary to widespread belief, *DO NOT* eat their way to fatness. Some people, just through the nature of life, are born to be fatter than what the media deems acceptable. How many of you know, deep in your heart, that you would have to starve yourself to reach media standards? How many of you exercise on a regular basis and eat a healthy diet and are still fatter than you believe is acceptable. How many of you are throwing your money into the diet industry's pockets and are not getting the results you were led to believe?

Have you ever tried a diet that "Guaranteed results or your money back"? Not a chance! The diet industry sets us up for failure and down deep we all know it. It's called hope. That one didn't work so I'll try this one. This one doesn't work so I'll try the other one. The other one didn't work so I'll go back to the one I tried years ago. All the emphasis on diets, a $50 billion industry, and North Americans are fatter than they have ever been. The only thing we lose when we buy into the next diet gimmick is money and self-esteem.

We need to stand up and recognize what the media deems natural is outrageous. If we were all meant to look like Kate Moss or Twiggy, clothes would not be made in sizes 16, 18 or 20. If we all had access to thousands of dollars to spend each day on hair, makeup, personal trainers, chefs, clothing connoisseurs, not to mention nip, tuck, suck, prick and implant, we would all look like the movie stars we are trying to emulate. Movie stars don't even need willpower—it is taken care of for them by their nutritionist, their personal trainer, their chauffeur, their maid and their masseuse. It's not real and it's not realistic.

"My weight consumes 70 per cent of my brain space."
Interview client #46

Look at your genetics, not the fashion industry.

We need to take a good hard look at our mothers and sisters and grandmothers. If your mother, grandmother and aunts are all shaped like Spartan apples with feet, there is a pretty good chance that you are going to be shaped like one too. We are genetically pre-programmed to be a certain body shape, weight range, body type and size—just like our foot size, hair color, eye color, and height. What do brunettes want? Blond hair. What do brown-eyed women want? Blue eyes. What do short women want to be? Tall. What do shy women want to be? Extroverted. What the hell is with wanting something that God didn't give you? Why can't you and I just say, "My body is a gift, just like my life is a gift, and I am going to do everything I can to take care of it"? Love *it*, for God's sake.

I interviewed many, many women for this book who truly believe that the key to happiness is thinness. It didn't matter if their husband was an alcoholic, they hated their job, their mother had cancer, they were in financial distress and they hadn't had a day off in three months, if they could just lose 20 pounds, everything else would be okay. Sound familiar?

"For me everything will be better when I am skinny. I will be happier and people will perceive me as a happier, more worthy person. Intimacy will be better. Life in general will be happier. I have felt since I was about 16 and still feel today, that when I am skinnier everything will change and my life will really start. I will be able to walk down the street happy and confident with my body. I know it is wrong but even though I am "happy" now....I feel real happiness will start when I lose the extra weight."   **Interview client #15**

"Society doesn't give you a chance to be okay with who you are before it comes along and says you need to look better."
                    Interview client #46

"Society doesn't value uniqueness."**Interview client #50**

We need to realize that very few women are gifted with a metabolism like a Porsche 911. Most women have a metabolism like a Pinto with a load of rocks in the back seat. We all have a pre-determined set-point but we spend our lives confusing it, which ultimately makes us fatter.

Set-point refers to our bodies internal desire to be and to remain at a healthy weight based on personal physiology. It is genetically pre-determined and is controlled by metabolic hormones and fat cell enzymes. It is part of our DNA, just like height and eye color. *You* may want to weigh 120 pounds but your body naturally wants to weigh 145 pounds. Be aware that if you fight your body's natural need to be 145 pounds, over time you will weigh 160 or 180 or 220 pounds because you keep damaging your genetic desire. Each time you go on a diet (DIE with a t) you restrict calories, (here is the part where you go yeah, yeah, I've heard it a million times). Your body recognizes this as a famine and slows your metabolism down in order to burn those restricted calories slower. You lose 10 pounds and start to eat normally again. Now you're eating with a metabolism like a Pinto with a load of rocks in the back seat *and* a flat tire. Not only are you carrying around those extra 10 pounds *again* but you've added a few more on top of that. Try doing that 30 or 40 times over 15 or 20 years and any logical person can see it is a recipe for disaster. Not only does yo-yo dieting eventually lead to a higher set-point, but it makes us fat and may lead to an eating disorder.

Every time we go on a calorie restricted Die with a t we re-establish our metabolism in order to accommodate our set-point. If you are finding no matter how hard you try to lose those last 10 pounds, they just won't come off, it is likely because your body is trying just as hard to hang on to those last 10 pounds because of your metabolism and natural set-point. This is why some people can eat and eat and eat and never gain weight. Their metabolism speeds up to accommodate the excess calories in order to maintain the natural set-point. The same holds true for those who have to watch everything they eat. They naturally have a slower metabolism that also wants to maintain a certain set-point.

Aim for progress not perfection.

We need to look at the psychological and cultural issues behind why we eat the way we do. Food is the one medication of choice that we can't just quit cold turkey because we need it to survive. Food is part of social gatherings such as birthdays, holidays, staffroom functions, weekends, friends for dinner, brunches, lunches out, camping and so on. Food is a socially acceptable medication for what ails us. Learning to recognize why we are eating, or more importantly overeating, is part of the key to our weight loss and weight management success. I have one dear friend who lost 40 pounds and one of the choices she made was to limit her alcohol intake to four ounces and very rarely any more. Well, she has four ounces—every night! She loves it, she enjoys it, she savors it, she looks forward to it, she sips it slowly. When it is gone, that is it. She made a commitment to herself and to her health, no one else and nothing else. It would be great if we could all learn from her example.

Next time you are invited to a birthday party, don't eat the whole cake! Have a thin piece and enjoy every bite of it. Going out for lunch? Pick something off the menu and clarify that you are doing it because you have made a choice to eat better not because, "I really should". Never-ending baking in the staff room? Find a different place to enjoy your lunch. Bored in the evening so you sit down in front of the television and eat the cardboard box that is left from the cookies you ate last night in front of the television? Why not get up and go for a walk, or have a bath or give yourself a pedicure or phone a friend. It is about conscious choices. Being present when you make the choice and being present when you eat the choice.

You are what you do.

In order to understand the dieting dilemma, we need to look at family patterns, family behaviors and family messages. When we are born, our diet is pre-determined by our parent's knowledge and lifestyle. If you were raised without breakfast or were allowed to leave the house without eating breakfast, chances are you are not going to be a breakfast eater. If you were raised by a mother that nurtured through baking, chances are you are going to associate baked goods with love and comfort. If you were given money every day to eat your school lunch at McDonald's, the chance of you being fatter and loving processed food is inevitable. Our dietary blueprint comes from our childhood and is determined by our upbringing, therefore it has to be a choice for us to change what we know, in order to learn something better. A habit to break.

A habit is an act so frequently repeated that it almost becomes automatic. If you look it up in the dictionary, it is also referred to as an addiction. It takes more than willpower and personal strength to break a habit, it takes a change in the way you think about the problem. You have to want the change with every inch of your being. Your desire to break the habit has to be stronger than the circumstances that keep the habit alive. You have to commit, with intention, to change.

Habits are things we do consciously and unconsciously such as shutting the bathroom door or brushing our teeth in the morning or eating breakfast or chewing our nails or eating when we are not hungry. Breaking a habit takes a continuous, conscious effort with a desire greater than that which causes the habit. It takes more than willpower to break a habit, it takes lifestyle changes. For example, not sitting in front of the television and consuming a whole tub of ice-cream takes a conscious decision to acknowledge why you want the ice-cream, why you want the whole tub of ice-cream and what you can do instead of eating the whole tub of ice-cream. It might be as simple as being conscious when you are eating or as difficult as having to find a professional to help you sort through what is causing you to eat when you are not hungry.

The problem with a habit is that it takes considerably less effort to create a habit than it does to break one. Take smoking as an example. Pretty easy to start smoking and to continue to smoke and to increase the amount you smoke, but very difficult to break the habit. Let's take an example that doesn't have to do with an addictive substance. A habit such as listening to the stereo in the car. If you're like me, it goes on before the heat or the air conditioning. Try driving in your car without the CD player on and notice how foreign and quiet and annoying it feels, but try to break the habit. Now let's take a habit as addictive, as socially acceptable and as emotionally charged as eating. That is a habit that takes major lifestyle changes to break. Lifestyle changes that affect all aspects of our lives from daily meals, social events, grocery shopping, and holidays, not to mention the emotional aspects such as past traumas and relationships.

Addictions are a loss of our soul.

Food is the most addictive substance available to us because we can't live without it. Learning to eat because we are hungry and learning to stop because we are full, is essential to breaking the habit. Learning that thin does not mean happiness and fat does not mean disgusting, is essential to breaking the habit. Learning to love the skin you are in and accepting what you were given, is essential to breaking the habit. Getting rid of the stressors that cause us to eat unconsciously and replace them with positive lifestyle changes, is essential to breaking the habit. Learning to stop eating our emotions is critical.

Addiction can be defined as—*The condition of being habitually or compulsively occupied with or involved in something.* For many women being thin is an addiction. I am not talking about the anorectic or the bulimic, I am talking about the average woman raising a family, holding down a job, going to aerobics class, having coffee with friends, who is constantly preoccupied with the concept of thin. She buys the fashion magazines, watches *America's Next Top Model*, buys everything low fat, reads *The South Beach* diet, *The Atkins* diet, *The Zone* diet, doesn't buy pants until the size goes down one, has the designer scale that weighs to the ounce, never weighs herself at night, dreams about being thin, keeps a medicine cabinet full of cellulite-cream, diet pills, and metabolic boosters, (Sound like you? Should I continue?). These are the addicted women I am talking about. Ask them if they have an eating disorder and they can honestly answer no. Ask them if they have a weight addiction and if they answer truthfully, the answer will be yes. If you think about the two addictions, the degree of separation between the two is thin enough to slide an ultra-slim, low-fat cheese slice through.

We as a society are consumed with, and addicted to, the concept of thin. We have done it to ourselves, we continue to do it to ourselves and will continue to do it to our ourselves and our children if we don't learn to accept and love our bodies. I will ask this question periodically throughout the book. Do you know a happy, thin women? Does she have everything you want or are her ribs just a little closer to the surface than yours? Is she wealthier than you or are all her dimples in her cheeks? Is she healthier than you or does her jean size mean she won't get cancer? Does her husband love her more because she can hang her skirt just right off her hip bones? Ridiculous? Yes. Instead of trying so hard to look like her, try to look like a better you.

Some women are born to be thin. I know you want to throw rocks at them, call them skinny bitches, hate them, *accidentally* trip them when they are leaving yoga class, and spread rumors that they are pregnant with the other skinny bitch's husband. Down deep we know it's because they have something that we want and don't have. Ask yourself, "Was I born to be thin? Is my mom thin? Are my siblings thin? Have I worked hard at my nutrition and my exercise? Do I eat consciously? Do I have a healthy relationship with food? Do I avoid diets and eat sensibly? Do I nurture myself and accept myself the way I am"? If you can honestly answer *yes* to all of these questions and you are still heavier than you want to be, perhaps it is time to accept that you were just meant to be a healthy, heavier person. It is also time to accept that we are what we do and we are what we eat and we are what we feel. If you want to change what you look like and how you feel, you have to change what you do and how you think.

Sticks and stones can break my bones but…..

One of the women I interviewed explained she was the youngest of five children and was born to older parents. Her mother believed that looking good was disobedient therefore she was not taught the basics of personal grooming. When she arrived in junior high she didn't understand anything about make-up, designer clothes or highlighted hair. She lacked self-esteem, and became the brunt of young boys' ruthless comments and actions. She remembers walking past groups of boys and they would comment, '10, 8.5, I'd do her, dog, -2, zero,

gross'. She knew she was the dog, the -2, and the gross.
Interview client #12

"I was camping and on the way back to the tent I was wearing a towel and one of the girls said, 'I'm surprised you can fit a towel around you'." **Interview client #40**

"I can remember being eight years old and waiting for the Sears catalogue so that I could get new clothes. When the catalogue finally came, my two girlfriends and I would sit down and circle the clothes we wanted. All the same because we were best friends. I remember one year when the clothes arrived, none of them fit me. I was two sizes bigger than my two friends and I was humiliated. From that point on I thought I was fat." **Interview client #20**

"When I was nine or 10 my mother used to serve dessert to everyone but me. She used to buy low fat milk for me and regular milk for everyone else because I was the chubby one."
Interview client #38

"I can remember when I was skating. I was told by a head coach in Skate Canada that I was too big for the sport and needed to lose weight. That was when I became conscious about my body." **Interview client #63**

"When I was in my teens, my brother used to call me a beached whale and I can still remember how much that bothered me."
Interview client #57

"I can recall very many 'single moments' when I felt people where whispering behind my back or just looking at me disdainfully." **Interview client #61**

Compared to what?

"I can't look at things the way they are without comparing them to myself and then I think, 'If I do that then people must be doing the same to me'." **Interview client #46**

"We compare ourselves because of all the magazines that have the thin, beautiful girls on them." **Interview client #63**

"Comparing comes from the expectations of ourselves and those around us. It also comes from everything that is pumped at us through the media." **Interview client #56**

"I constantly compare because of the images that surround us that reinforce the idea that looking good equals happiness."
Interview client #51

"I thinks it's because we always want what we don't have."
Interview client #32

What is it that causes us to constantly compare ourselves to others? Is it the need to feel superior? As long as I look better than you, you can be my friend. As long as you are fatter than me, I will be your friend. As long as I am richer than you, you can be my friend. I wish I looked like so and so. I wish I had a nicer car than so and so. I wish our house was as big as so and so. I wish my career was as exciting as so and so. I wish I could afford to dress like so and so. Meanwhile, we spend so much time comparing ourselves to so and so that we never take the time to enjoy who we are and what we have. Time ticks on.

You may say, "Well you don't know what it is like to be fat or to be broke or to be made fun of or to drive a shitty car." I say, "Who cares!" Who cares if someone is skinnier, richer, taller, more successful, drives a nicer car, or wears nicer clothes? Does that make them a better person? Does that mean they are happy? Does that mean they don't compare themselves to other skinnier, richer, more successful people? Does that mean they won't get cancer? Does that mean if you had those things you would be happy? It's a self-defeating game, just like dieting.

Why not accept that, in many ways, we have created the life we live and if we are not happy with the life we are living, comparing and judging are not going to change it? Only you can change it and I believe starting with yourself is the key. If we could only learn to accept our strengths and weaknesses as just that, strengths and weaknesses, maybe we would begin to capitalize on our strengths and work on our weaknesses, in order to make *our* life a better life. The key to change begins with our attitude. Believing that you're not too fat, would be a great place to start.

2
SELF-DESTRUCTION

It is sad knowing there are people in the world that are suffering so badly they are willing to self-destruct. That is to destroy oneself by choice. There are many ways that people choose to self-destruct but the one that is important to this book is the self-destructive habit of dieting and weight loss. It's ironic at the same time we are living, we are slowly dying. Some people are just speeding up the process.

"When I first started to self-destruct it began with sleeping in my running clothes. I would get up at 4 a.m. and run and run and run and then get back into bed before my parents got up so they wouldn't know. Next I began to live on salads, then slowly started to omit everything from my diet. I read a book that listed all the *free foods*, meaning foods that had no calories. I eventually structured my entire diet around those foods."

Interview client #5

"I wanted to die but I was afraid of pain so driving into a tree wasn't an option. I was afraid of the sight of blood so slitting my wrists wasn't an option. I didn't do drugs and there were none in the house so an overdose wasn't an option. So I decided to starve myself to death because it seemed less messy and maybe no one would notice." **Interview client #12**

"I was committed to the psyche ward, the first time, by my mother and my family doctor, at the age of 18. When I spoke to the counselor I told him I thought I had an eating disorder but he didn't listen and asked why I was depressed. It was a weird, crazy place that had no idea how to deal with an eating-disordered patient who didn't *look* eating-disordered. I drank nothing but tea for two weeks and no one, not even the nurses, noticed because I didn't look eating-disordered. Eventually I walked out of the psyche ward with a psychotic, schizophrenic that I became mixed up with. Once we were out and he left me because I was so messed up, I slit my wrists and took a bunch of pills. My father found me and I was once again shipped back to the psyche ward. I was eventually referred to a psyche ward in Vancouver. This was the second time, there were more to come." **Interview client #22**

Die with a t

Dieting can be as self-destructive to our self-esteem and our health as drugs and alcohol. We use diets as a way to tell ourselves that we are not okay the way we are. Diets, dysfunctional eating and eating disorders can be very seductive. Like a romance novel, diets (DIE with a t) lead us to believe a story that is not true. When we diet we think everything in life will be better. We will get a better job. Our husband will love us more. Our friends will look up to us. We will get rich, our mobile home will turn into a 10,000 square foot mansion and our fat husband will, poof, look like Brad Pitt. Our flea infested dog will turn into a pure bred Maltese with a diamond studded collar, our pot-smoking teenagers will join a gospel choir and our Pinto will turn into a Porsche 911. I was amazed at the number of women I interviewed who truly believed that weight loss was the answer to all their problems. Truly believed— without any question or hesitation, poof—happiness. Do you believe that?

"At first I felt like I was in control of everything. Calories in and calories out, down to the minute detail. Files, books, journals. Eventually I lost control and *it* took over."

Interview client #7

Do you believe that thin means goodness, morality, happiness and success and that fatness means badness, immorality, unhappiness and a lack of success? Stop and look around you. I mean really stop and look around. What does the head female teller at your bank look like? What does the female owner of your favorite restaurant look like? What do 90 per cent of the women at your gym look like? What do 90 per cent of the women on the beach look like? What does your best friend look like? What do the middle-age women driving the big expensive cars look like? Like you? Some maybe not, but most, yes. Why are we self-destructing our minds, our values, our bodies and our self-esteem to look like something only a small portion of society looks like and very often looks like at the expense of their physical and mental health? Why can't we see that what we are trying so desperately to become is a false-self, riddled with all the same ironies, self-doubt, frustration, anger, and pain—just in a smaller body?

I recently watched a television show called the *Vanity Insanity*. It was about a woman who became addicted to plastic surgery at a very young age, filling her face full of saline to plump it, pout it, and enhance it. Not knowing the consequences of having a foreign substance injected into her face, she continued having the procedures done because she loved the way it made her look. Slowly over time the saline injections started to seep and pool and created pockets and pouches which wrapped around nerve endings and created facial paralysis and disfigurement. At the time of the special she looked to be about 60 and had had over 50 surgeries, both enhancement and reconstructive. She looked horribly disfigured but had no intention of stopping. She said until she was in her casket she wanted to look beautiful.

We all want to look beautiful and feel attractive but at what expense? Are you willing to commit *silent suicide* to look thin? Are you willing to vomit into Ziplock baggies and hide them in the clothes hamper to look thin? Are you willing to alienate your friends and family to be thin? Are you willing to risk your health to look thin? Are you willing to risk your marriage, your job, your relationships to look thin?

Everyone's dying but not everyone's living.

Self-destruction comes in many forms. We can self-destruct our finances, our relationships, our health, our happiness, our bodies, our children, our lives. We do it with alcohol, gambling, drugs, sex, money, work, food or any combination of these vices. At the heart of every self-destructive soul is an alter ego trying just as hard to survive—it's called *self-preservation*.

Over the years I have learned just how systematically the body will shut down in order to survive. This can be illustrated with a disease as serious as anorexia, where the body is forced to *eat* it's own organs in order to hang on just a little longer. It can also be illustrated with a simple example such as weight loss versus fat loss. The body hangs onto the fat for self-preservation. The metabolism slows down in order to burn fewer calories, slower, for self-preservation. Our energy level decreases in order to accommodate the metabolic decrease to ensure self-preservation. Whatever it takes to survive is what the body inherently knows how to do.

Sometimes having more fat than we would like, is what is programmed into our DNA survival map. If we spend our lives trying to negate what we were pre-determined to be, you can only image the consequences. It would be like putting regular gas in a diesel engine or walking on a broken leg or living on processed food. You may get away with it for a period of time but eventually you'll pay the price.

Diets are one of the most socially acceptable ways to destroy our self-esteem and our health. The media promotes it. Our mothers participate in it. Our doctors recommend it. Our health clubs encourage it. Our role models sponsor it. Our society loves it. Imagine if women didn't diet—they wouldn't have anything to talk about! It has become such a normal way of life for women that it is going to take some serious brainwashing for women to accept that diets don't work. In order for women to accept and admit that diets don't work, they have to admit that the only alternative to dieting, for weight loss, is hard work, patience and personal acceptance. If they admit that diets don't work, they have to give up hope that the next one will be the answer. As long as there is another diet out there or another quick fix then there will be hope for the eternal fountain of thinness. If they admit diets don't work, they will feel as though there is no hope for their dream of becoming thin.

It is time to stop self-destructing. Start self-educating instead. The more you know about how your body reacts every time you restrict calories, the better the chance you will stop the pattern. The sooner you understand that fad diets are not the answer, that a change in lifestyle is, the sooner you get to start living. The more you understand that moving burns calories, the more motivated you are going to be to move.

Pain

Women caught on the diet treadmill, with no emergency stop button, have many things in common. Despair, frustration, fear, anger, and pain. The pain of being trapped in a body they don't want and don't know how to get out of. The pain of feeling less than acceptable because the media implies that thin is the only way to be perfect. The pain of feeling disgusting. The pain of being judged. The pain of being criticized. The pain of being laughed at. So what then is pain? In this case it is mental suffering. It is the kind of pain we medicate with food and patch up with diets. It is the kind of pain that can't be healed with aspirins, band-aids or Echinacea. Food is our aspirin and diets are our band-aids.

We know that walking on a bed of burning coals will burn our feet and cause excruciating pain so we don't do it. We know that jumping off a ten-storey building will cause severe road rash so we don't do it. We know that hitting ourselves on the head with a cast iron pan will give us a bad headache so we don't do it. If you knew how much pain dieting would cause you when you got older, would you still have done it? If you know how much pain it will cause your daughter if she begins to diet, will you do everything you can to educate her on how destructive diets can be? You have that opportunity. It's not too late.

My Story:

I have spent so much of my life hating my body
and waiting/weighting for the day that the
wait/weight will be over and off.
Well that day has never magically dis/appeared
and I am still waiting/weighting.
I have put off being happy, put off knowing
my own voice but kept putting on the weight
and the loneliness. I isolated myself and
my pain into my hatred of my fat.
I ate to not feel and slept to not be conscience
of the hatred that consumed my body.

Sarah Kerr
Professional Photographer
Courtenay, B.C.

"When I was about 40 my husband and I were trying to make love except he couldn't get an erection, he said it was because I was too fat and didn't arouse him. It was then that I threw up my hands and said I don't care anymore and came out of the closet as a closet eater and slowly ate my way to 220 pounds."
Interview client #22

"Last summer I was back east and decided to attend my 30th high school reunion. My old boyfriend from high school and my close friends were all going to be there. I spoke to a few of them over the phone and decided to go. When I arrived only one of my friends could look me in the eye and I knew it was because I had gained so much weight. I remember my friends saying that I was always the pretty one, the skinny one, the popular one and now no one would have anything to do with me. As my friend and I were leaving, my old boyfriend offered to give us a ride home. When we got to the car, his wife—whom I also went to school with—said, 'Now is your chance. Do you want to take him out back of the barn for one more roll in the hay?' She had no idea how badly that hurt because I know that if I was still slim and pretty, she never would have made that offer but because I wasn't, I was safe."

Interview client #22

"Dysfunctional eating is my best friend! I know what to expect from it. It's mine and I own it in a life that seems so out of control."

Interview client #20

Rock bottom

Have you ever noticed that a good diet always starts on Monday? You eat your way through the weekend knowing full well that Sunday night is going to be the last supper. Monday morning rolls around and you are motivated by great intentions, then your girlfriend phones you in distress and asks if you can join her for lunch at her favorite bakery, for her favorite distress meal and all your great intentions seem to be gladly forgotten until next Monday.

"I really hit rock bottom when my kids were little and I have been fighting ever since. I got involved with the Overeater's Anonymous program the summer of 2003 and I learned a lot about my disease and that I am not alone. It means though that I must work a very disciplined program and stay within that support system. I haven't as much lately and I see myself slipping. I think joining my gym helped. I feel safe there. I see all kinds of body shapes and I am starting to see that being healthy and happy does not mean you have to be thin. I have learned to put more emphasis on my fitness and less on how I look. Being strong and being able to do spin class has been my goal. I love the friendly atmosphere and I like that I know people and have developed small friendships. It keeps me going. This is what I need. I need to get out of the mind-set of being thin and exercise because I feel better for it. It is the social and fun aspect of exercise that keeps me going."

Interview client #12

"We always knew she would have to hit *rock bottom* before she would ever *come out*, and that is what happened this summer, in June. Since then, every day has been a struggle......for us parents the emotional struggle is unbearable at times, and I sometimes wonder if we will make it through this. Professionals tell us that we have to take a step back and let her battle this on her own, along with her support group consisting of a fabulous family physician, a nutritionist and a clinical therapist. She has been in hospital 18 times with extremely low potassium, sometimes ending up in telemetry, hooked up to heart monitors etc., with potassium levels down to 2.1. There were mornings when I just couldn't open her bedroom door to see if she was still breathing, and had to ask my husband to check on her." **Mother**

"I hit rock bottom when I was taking a class at Ron Zalko's and Ron asked me if I was going to be okay. I slid down the wall with blue lips as I was consuming nothing but Diet Coke."

Interview client #36

Sometimes the best things that happen to us are the worst situations. They provide the greatest opportunity for change. They become our epiphanies, our fork in the road, our motivation for change. It may be an alcoholic that causes a serious car accident that kills a child because they were drinking and driving. A woman who develops skin cancer because of an obsession with being tanned. The end of a marriage because of an eating disorder. Bankruptcy because of a gambling addiction. Whatever the story may be, the situation has to become more unbearable than that which caused the situation in the first place. Discomfort is a prime motivator. Harrison Ford once said, "You have to have a darkness for the dawn to come."

For you, maybe your rock bottom is not so drastic but eventually you are going to have to admit that living on the diet treadmill is not living and being overweight is not dying and getting off of the diet treadmill and being a little overweight is at least a start at life. Acceptance. Lifestyle change. Motivation. Success.

"I have had many rock bottoms. The hardest was when my depression became so deep that I began actively looking for someone to take my kids because I knew I would not be alive much longer. I wished every day that I would not wake up in the morning."   **Interview client #42**

"The weigh scale was like a gauge to determine just how wrong things were in my life."   **Interview client #39**

When I asked women what their rock bottom was, some could answer without hesitation but many felt they still hadn't hit rock bottom or they wouldn't still be suffering. I believe that every diet is another rung on the ladder leading to rock bottom. The problem is, there is a never-ending supply of diets, therefore you may be on the longest ladder known to man! Either hang on and attempt a fireman's exit so you can hit rock bottom and get it over with or look up and start climbing out of the weight loss pit. Look at each rung as a step toward your goal and away from rock bottom. Don't worry if you slip or fall, just start climbing back up again. Eventually, you'll see the light.

entrapped

numb
numb to any feeling or emotions
numb to my own words
      my own thoughts
            my own voice
and I am alone
      in the confinement
            of this mental cage
                  in which this monster
is holding me
      making me feel this way
feel numb
there is no way out
no escape
no door, no window
nothing
he holds me here
      day and night
and he will for the rest of my life
for the rest of every
      hour, minute, second
he terrorizes me
      he teases me
            he puts pictures into my head
the one I must listen to
for eternity
because there is no escaping
      yourself.......

Interview client #7

3
DESPERATION

As an intelligent, highly-motivated, multi-tasking, determined, courageous breed, it is astounding that women would fall for an eating plan that sells us dehydrated food in cryovac packages that arrive bubble wrapped in a box from the other side of the country. Mmmmm, that sounds so yummy I think I'll join! What about the tea that dissolves belly fat or the one that tells us that 60 per cent of our nutrition should come from fat. That diet is going to be highly successful—in terms of people becoming more fat. My favorite is the one that states: a shake for breakfast, a shake for lunch and a "sensible" meal for dinner. Well, after a shake for breakfast and a shake for lunch, a side of beef and a bag of potatoes is going to be a "sensible" dinner—along with the pot they were cooked in.

Our brain's main source of energy comes from carbohydrates, which are broken down into glucose. The term *fat head* makes no sense but *potato head* sure does. If we don't fuel our brain, it doesn't function properly. If we deprive ourselves of carbohydrates on an ongoing basis, our perception becomes skewed. Our ability to think straight, to focus, to rationalize and to react appropriately becomes compromised. Think about those diets that tell us that too many carbohydrates make us fat, therefore we should cut our carbohydrate consumption back to almost nothing. What do you think is the first thing to become compromised? Our ability to think clearly and to rationalize. We develop those lovely mood swings, total confusion, a wee bit of anger all wrapped up in a nice little ball of depression. This can be especially true for women who suffer from anorexia. It is normal for a healthy mind to observe an anorectic and wonder why she can't see how painfully skinny she is, how awful she looks or why she just won't eat but *their* minds have suffered from malnourishment for so long that their reality comes from a starving brain.

When we starve our bodies, especially with low carbohydrate diets, our brain interprets this as a famine and becomes obsessed with food. Ever notice when you say the word diet, you automatically start thinking about your next meal or snack or the bakery down the street or the stale crackers in the cupboard? Combine this with mood swings, irritability, confusion and depression and then ask yourself—is this worth it? Is this worth it or would I be happier a bit heavier with normal eating habits? Would my husband and children enjoy being around me because I'm not such a bitch? Would I stop being obsessed with food if I just started eating it the way it was meant to be eaten? Eat when you're hungry, stop when you're full.

An important point to understand about food and our body is the way carbohydrates and fats work together to produce an efficient energy burning system. Without carbohydrates, which get converted to glucose in our bodies, we cannot burn fat effectively. Think about carbohydrates as the kindling that starts the fire burning in our muscles and fat as the giant logs that keep the fire burning for long, slow periods of time. Without both, you either have a fire that dies out very quickly, or one that won't start.

Do you know a happy skinny woman?

One of the many women interviewed for this book was a beautiful, tall, blonde mother of two that had a body like a model but suffered her entire life with eating disorders. When I asked her to comment on some of the crazy rituals or diets she had embarked on, I was surprised by how easily the memories came back to her. She stole food. She took laxatives and forced herself to vomit. She lied about food. She felt like cutting herself so she would feel any pain other than the pain in her head. She felt like killing herself. She lashed out at others and hurt so many people because of her pain. She spent days locked away at home eating non-stop until she fell into a sugar-high-drunken-stupor that could only be slept off. She let the disease control her life. Being thin was the most important thing in her life and it took priority over her two children, her husband and her job. When asked what she lost along the way, she stated, "Life's experiences because I wasn't perfect enough to do them." Her desperation to be thin was her sole purpose. She had no concept of what too thin was or what happiness meant.

Women have a tendency to confuse thinness with happiness. While interviewing for this book, I met very few thin women who didn't feel much the same as the women who wanted to lose 50 pounds. I think we do these women a disservice by assuming happiness or unhappiness based on size.

Their desperation to be thin is sometimes masked as thin. Being ultra-thin is very often a desperate measure to hide or to disappear. Women I spoke to that had suffered from eating disorders or were currently suffering from eating disorders spoke a common language of desperation.

"I love to be very thin. I love to hear I am too thin. I like my clothes to feel loose. I feel more feminine and sexy. I feel more energetic. I feel that I can handle more of life's stressors if I am thin. If I am thin, I am attractive and then no matter what else happens in my life, I have that. I have something that others want and it is a safeguard. People like beautiful people. They are drawn to them." **Interview client #12**

"When I was really, really thin, I was really happy with my body but not with myself. That is when I realized the two don't go together." **Interview client #74**

Many times when we judge women by their appearance it is because the appearance is not deemed socially acceptable. For example, a woman who is 40 pounds overweight enjoying a burger and fries at the food court at the local mall. You may look at her and say she is fat, therefore she must be unhappy. But maybe she has been 40 pounds overweight for 20 years and is completely content. Maybe this is her once a month treat. The opposite scenario holds true. You may look at a beautiful prima ballerina, making a living doing what she loves more than anything in life. A waif with the grace and beauty of a butterfly dying inside because she's not quite thin enough.

Because we are living in such an image-based society, we are constantly inundated with images designed to sell us on a product or a concept. Unfortunately products all use the same belief to sell them and the belief is that thin is the perfect ideal. You never see an ad with a fat woman selling perfume or a fat woman selling jeans or a fat woman selling a car. Because we are constantly bombarded with the image of skinny we begin to think it is the norm or the ideal and if you don't fit into the ideal, you are free game for judgment and ridicule. Judgment and ridicule were the two most painful consequences of being fat. In the video, *A Matter of Fat*, written and produced by Antony Thomas for CBC, a class of children ranging in ages from five to eight were each given four pictures. The first picture was a child with no hair from radiation therapy, the second was a child from a unique ethnic background, the third was a child in a wheelchair and the fourth was a fat boy. The children were asked to look at the photos and pick the photo of the one child they did *not* want to be their friend. The children overwhelmingly picked the picture of the fat boy. He was picked more than the other three combined. When the children were asked why they had picked that boy they said it was because he was fat. When asked why they thought he was fat, they all said it was because he was lazy.

I'm starving!

I listen to women talking about weight loss, even bragging about it, every single day. The common line, "I'm starving", used as though they had any idea what starving really felt like. A total lack of regard for those living in true famine. Women tossing around how little they eat as though it were a badge of honor. "I never eat breakfast, I never eat lunch, I never eat fast food, I rarely eat supper, salad only for supper, I don't eat on Tuesdays, I don't eat when I get my period, I don't eat on Saturdays or Fridays for that matter, I never eat on a full moon, when it's sunny, when it's raining, when I've had a massage."

It is important to realize when we diet or restrict food intake for long periods of time, our brains become obsessed with food. Many of you have experienced this scenario—you commit to starting a new diet on Monday and when it rolls around, all you can think about is food. Keep in mind that our brains exist off glucose, so the longer we go limiting our calories, especially carbohydrates, the more disoriented we become—and bitchy, and crabby, and frustrated, and so on and so on. Malnutrition also causes a chemical imbalance in the brain which can lead to eating disorders. What someone initially intended as a weight loss program, with no history of mental illness, if left to progress too far could become an eating disorder. We were not meant to restrict our food intake to meager portions just like we were not meant to eat until we felt as though we would vomit. Food is meant to be a fuel that allows us to complete our activities of daily life. Maybe if we are lucky and have developed a healthy relationship with food, we can even enjoy it along the way. We were not meant to manipulate it, hide it, abuse it, hate it or fear it. Food is a gift just like our life and our bodies. If we lived in parts of Africa or India we would think so.

Controlling the uncontrollable.

One of the many wonderful women that I interviewed had a trunk full of Pearls of Wisdom from her food journey. She was a constant stream of ironies. One of her most profound ironies was her ability to control her purging seizures.

Whenever she was genuinely sick with the flu she would have to be very careful to have people around her because if she became sick to her stomach, she would suffer from seizures. It was a medical condition. When she was at the height of her bulimia, getting sick several times a day, she knew exactly what could happen when she purged but she did it anyway because she knew *she* was controlling the purging, therefore *she* was controlling the seizures. Her desperation to be thin was her sole purpose.

Desperation—*the recklessness that grows out of despair.* After researching for this book, I truly believe that diets (DIE with a t) are a desperate measure to become something other than what you are. Society has made you feel that who you are is not good enough. How many of you reading this book have been on diets since your mother told you she loved your chubby little butt? How many of you, while reading this book, are wondering why Mr. Christie and his good friend Ding Dong, keep calling your name from the cupboard? How many of you can justify that carrot cake is a "healthy treat" because it has the word carrot in it? What about eating too much last night so I just won't eat today? Desperate.

Desperation comes from feeling like you have no options and that life is impossible. "My husband will never love me the way I love him," munch, munch, munch. "I'll never get the job that I applied for," munch, munch, munch. "My mother never thinks I'm good enough," munch, munch, munch. "I can't see past my shitty life," munch, munch, munch. "If I could only catch a break," munch, munch, munch. "It's impossible to lose weight so why try," munch, munch, munch. And out of desperation you munch your way to fatness. Baseball Hall of Fame recipient, Tommy Lasorda once said, "The difference between the impossible and the possible lies in a person's determination". Women should start to yoga their way to fitness, walk their way to clarity, bathe their way to calmness, and laugh their way to happiness.

"I told my teachers in school that I just wanted to pass. I didn't care how well I did and would only do what I absolutely had to do to pass. I didn't want to be in school because I was too busy playing with my eating disorder. I would make myself too busy so that I didn't have to eat and I would purposely overeat so that I could enjoy the feeling of throwing up."

Interview client #12

Desperate times call for desperate measures.

Insomnia is an interesting symptom of eating disorders and dysfunctional eating. I interviewed women who developed insomnia because their body was so afraid to shut down in case it died in its sleep. I interviewed women who developed chronic insomnia because of chemical imbalances and would average no more than three hours of sleep a night, for years. I also spoke with women who would not sleep because during sleep, very few calories were burned, therefore the longer they could stay awake each day, the more calories they were able to burn by the end of the week. Desperation.

Listening to so many women has taught me that sometimes the concept of life is just too much. It wasn't what they dreamed it would be and it isn't what they wanted it to be. Where was the romance, the fun, the spontaneity, the 'me' time, the love, and the certainty? I asked if the void they were trying to fill with food was a void of certainty or uncertainty. They would respond by saying, "The certainty that this is as good as it gets and the uncertainty that life would never get any better".

Debt, kids, divorce, marriage, death, illness, work, competition, media, wanting, needing. Regardless, life is what you have been presented with and it is what you make of it. Spend the rest of your life thinking about something other than your weight and body and you may find that you have the much needed energy to improve the qualities of your life that make you feel uncertain.

"I wish I didn't have to try so hard to be perfect."
Interview client #38

"I never got sick at school. No one ever saw me overeat. I played with my eating disorder in my basement where no one could see me or hear me." **Interview client #38**

"I was on a very strict diet of sweets."
Interview client #28

"I would go for a six hour walk and take one apple cut into slices. I would eat one slice every two hours."
Interview client #28

"If I had to explain to you all of the crazy ways I have tried to lose weight, well that would become a whole other book."
Interview client #21

"I was so desperate for positive affirmation that I forced myself to walk naked in front of my friend but felt crushed when he didn't respond." **Interview client #62**

"The process of trying to lose weight made me so unhappy I decided that being fat was better than being unhappy."
Interview client #47

"When I was in Grade 9 or 10, I was slightly anorexic. I would only eat enough items in a day to list on one hand. That was how I accounted for my daily food intake."
Interview client #46

"Sometimes in my life there has not been an hour in the day that I have not been thinking about my weight."
Interview client #60

"I know it isn't supposed to be, but somewhere in me I'm wanting to be thin more than anything else in the world."
Interview client #44

"At one point I was throwing up eight to 10 times per day. I had several occasions where I threw up blood for as long as two weeks at a time." **Interview client #42**

"My weight will always be a struggle and sometimes I don't have the energy to fight." **Interview client #27**

"I thought I would never get through a day without thinking about food—what/where/how/why/vomit."
Interview client #22

"I looked in the mirror and my eyes were dead."
Interview client #12

Life is more amusing than we think.

The scale is a tool designed to tell us the weight of a particular object. It can be black with tiger prints, or pink with a fuzzy cover, steel and gleaming, or clinical white. Regardless, it is still a scale and its job is to weigh what is put on it. When we weigh a banana, the scale doesn't know if it is a diamond or a hunk of coal or a banana. All it knows is how much it weighs. When we weigh the banana, the banana doesn't hold its breath in utter anticipation of what kind of day it is going to be— great if I am an ounce lighter than my other banana friend or miserable if I am an ounce heavier than I was yesterday. We are the only animals on the face of the Earth that allow the outcome of our day to be determined by a spring-loaded mechanism that lies on the bathroom floor with the dust bunnies and pubic hair.

But don't take it out on the scale if it doesn't show you what you want to see. Don't jump on it and yell at it and scream, "You don't know what you are talking about!" Give it a break, it is only doing its job—weighing what stands on it. It doesn't care how much water you drank this week or how little bread you ate or how well you abstained from your peanut butter and chocolate chip sandwiches. It doesn't recognize if you are the same person that stood on it yesterday, if you have your bum thong on, if you were nice to your neighbor or if you have your fingers crossed. All it knows is how much you weigh—fat, muscle, bone, water, organs, irrelevant. If you have become a slave to the scale it is time to realize that the greatest use of a bathroom weigh scale is to see how well it flies at 110 kilometers per hour while driving down the Inland Island Highway on your way to Mexico with your new bikini and your extra 18 pounds of fat. Just make sure you clean up the parts after it lands.

When I spoke with the young girls from various schools, I asked how many of them weighed themselves. Although not all the girls admitted to weighing, it did start as young as Grade 5 and Grade 6. At this age, there were quite a few of the girls that weighed themselves but it was interesting to note when I asked why they weighed themselves, they said they didn't really know why but that it was fun. I had a couple of young girls tell me that they liked to weigh themselves, then do a bunch of exercise and weigh themselves again. Almost all of the high school girls admitted to weighing themselves to make sure they weren't getting fat.

Kids should not be weighing themselves. There is absolutely no need for it unless they are extremely overweight. It is a self-defeating game that has no rules.

If an inanimate object, such as a scale, has the power to produce such a profound, negative effect on your body image and self-esteem, maybe it would be a good idea to get rid of it. If you have daughters and you know how poisoning a scale can be, perhaps you can prolong their curiosity by simply not having one.

"I weigh myself once a month or so—unless I am bored in which case I weigh myself a few times an hour."
Grade 8 student

"Yes, I weigh myself because it is fun."   **Grade 7 student**

"I weigh myself because it is fun and I think I am fat."
Grade 7 student

"I weigh myself all the time since we got a scale for Christmas."
Grade 7 student

"I weigh myself every second day because I want to lose weight."   **Grade 7 student**

As wonderfully intelligent women, regardless of size, we have become a slave to this little beast. Hoping every day it will tell us what society deems is the perfect weight, therefore size, therefore body. What the hell is the perfect body anyway? Can someone please enlighten me because after months of research, I still can't figure it out. Is it 5 foot 10, 125 pounds with a C cup or is it 5 foot 7, 118 pounds and an ass like a dancer? Is it 5 feet tall, 90 pounds, and a size five foot or is it Jennifer

Aniston or is it Angelina Jolie or is it Sophia Loren or is it Marilyn Monroe? Is it broad shoulders, is it narrow hips, is it a big booty, is it a small booty, is it big breasts, is it small breasts? Or, is it anything but what we are?

4

SIMPLE WEIGHT LOSS INFORMATION

Okay, let's establish some simple rules that some of you may know but don't understand and some of you may not know at all. I believe that any person who achieves their goals, regardless of what the goals are, does so by understanding each and every step required. Someone who decides they want to run a marathon will do so successfully if they take the appropriate training steps. In order to take the appropriate training steps, one must educate themselves about how to take each step and why, in order to avoid injury and failure. I developed a back care program several years ago and I believe part of the success of the program was the 45 minutes spent at the beginning of each course educating participants about the physiology and the mechanics of the spine. They were able to take the physiological information and apply it to each exercise and each stretch in order to understand why they were doing each one. This made it much easier for the participants to be compliant because they actually understood what would happen to their spine if they did the exercises and stretches incorrectly, aggressively or not at all. Education equals empowerment.

Your weight loss success depends on understanding how your body reacts to the nutritional abuse it is subjected to. Likewise, it will be easier to convince yourself of the importance of getting off the diet treadmill if you understand why diets are so destructive. Let's start with a real basic issue— breakfast. For those of you who have never noticed, the word breakfast, broken down, is break fast. Break-the-fast. Last night you had supper at 7 p.m. and then at 9 p.m. you downed a super size bowl of popcorn riddled with M & M's while watching *Desperate Housewives*. Off to bed you go at 10 p.m. amidst a sugar high and a sodium infusion, to flip and flop throughout the night dreaming it's raining Skittles. You wake up at 6:30 a.m. make yourself a cup of coffee and begin the drudgery of another day, committed to eating nothing but salads. You get the kids off to school, lunches made, permission slips signed, grocery list in hand, purse over one shoulder, briefcase under the other arm. You get to work just in time to refill your coffee cup and get caught up on the latest diet gossip. Off to your desk you go, cup in hand, while visions of a six pack of Big Macs (hold the mayo), from McDonald's swirl around in your head. Twelve phone calls and two reports later, the 10:30 a.m. coffee break saves the day. Off you go to refill your cup with a bit more caffeine to help stave off the fatigue you are feeling. The staff room is full of baking that has been banished from the kitchens of the diet slaves and ordered to be consumed by those skinny people. But you're not having any part of it—yet. Back to the desk you go, three more reports and a dozen e-mails. Feeling a bit light headed? Good thing lunch is around the corner.

By the time this woman finally eats lunch (assuming she eats lunch), she hasn't eaten since 9 p.m. the night before.

That was 15 hours ago. Do you ever go 15 hours during the day without eating? Then why would you do it, on a regular basis, regardless if it includes your sleep time? Your metabolism is like a muscle and she just committed metabolic sabotage! The more you work it, the fitter it gets; the less you work it, the more depressed it becomes, and trust me, you can't fix that depression with counseling. It is ironic that we have to eat in order to lose weight, isn't it? Break-the-fast is the most important meal of the day because it starts your metabolism working. It fires it up and forces it out of hibernation. Every time you feed it you force it to work. Keep in mind that what you feed it is just as important as feeding it.

"I really like my sleep, so I get up as late as possible, feed my kids, make their lunches, get them out the door, get myself out the door (without eating!), do a million things, come home at lunch, feed the three year old while continuing to do a million things (don't eat lunch), go on my computer and have a Pepsi and usually some chocolate at 1:30 p.m. Continue to do a million things and finally eat supper at 6 p.m.!"
Interview Client #30

Sugar is better than sex!

We know that sugar and fat are the two ingredients that make food taste so utterly desirable that we can't resist their sneaky little voices chanting, "Eat me, chew me, hide me." They intoxicate our senses and suffocate our willpower. They cause intelligent women to break down and kneel before the brownie pulpit nodding furiously as Mr. Christie baptizes another disciple in canola oil because it is unsaturated!

When I was organizing the panel discussions for the schools, I sat in one of the staff rooms with a counselor going over the logistics of the project and I was intrigued by the activity that took place. As I sat discussing guidelines for the project, women would float in and out and participate in the discussion. They would fill us in on their experiences with weight gain and diets and how it affects young girls these days, all the while consuming the cookies and pizza that had been brought into the staff room on that particular day. There were complaints, amidst the snacking, about how difficult it is to lose weight and how people just don't understand.

When we consume foods that are high in sugar and fat, our body breaks the food down into various components and places them in very specific spots. Fats circulate in the bloodstream and are eventually stored in fat cells hopefully to be burned off. Sugar circulates in the bloodstream and is stored in the liver and the muscles, hopefully to be burned off. For simplicity we will stick with these two nutrients. In small amounts, our body requires and thrives off fat and sugar. Unfortunately, small amounts is the problem.

When we consume larger than required amounts of sugar, our brain signals the pancreas to secrete insulin. Insulin is meant to keep our blood sugar at a manageable level. When there is too much sugar circulating, the insulin "grabs it by the hand" and brings it back down to a normal level. This little relationship works all day long without us knowing, regardless of how badly we abuse it. That is, of course, until we develop diabetes.

Now what happens when we have a surge of insulin circulating around in our body after a sugar feast? When the body has an excess of insulin circulating in the bloodstream, it opens the flood gates to the fat cells, which are sitting there saying, "Fill me up baby, cause I still got room!" Insulin is like the creepy gatekeeper in one of Stephen King's horror stories. It unlocks the door to the fat cells, takes the fat circulating in the bloodstream by the hand, and personally escorts it into the fat cells. Take something as delicious as a doughnut and you just provided that relationship with the perfect environment for fat storing. A piece of cake, if you'll pardon the pun. Fat and sugar combined equals pancreas, insulin, the gatekeeper and really, really happy fat cells. Cookies, Dairy Queen Blizzards, pies, cakes, doughnuts, chocolate bars, Pop-Tarts, and so on are perfect little fat storing demons, especially if you combine them with a high-sugar drink such as pop, sugary coffee drinks, alcohol and fruit drinks.

Although there does not appear to be a consistent RDA for sugar, the Official US Guideline recommends no more than 40 grams of sugar per day based on a 2,000 calorie diet. Depending on what type of sugar and how full the teaspoon is, one teaspoon of sugar is equal to approximately 4.5-5 grams, therefore a 2,000 calorie diet would allow for no more than eight to nine teaspoons of sugar per day. This is any form of sugar. If you're not sure what is considered a sugar, review the list of different forms of sugar under 'Reading labels' on page 62. Depending which website you read, a can of Pepsi contains approximately 10 teaspoons of sugar. A Sunkist Orange Soda contains 13 teaspoons and a glazed doughnut contains approximately six teaspoons of sugar.

Fat is the fast food industry's gift to the human race.

Fat is considered an essential nutrient—unfortunately not the amount we consume on a daily basis. Back in the simple days of the cavemen, when fashion wasn't an issue and neither were breast implants, pay-per-view, Botox, cheese-stuffed wieners or super size me, we ate out of necessity and we ate what was available off the land. There was no strange man with big red feet and very dated yellow pajamas skipping around handing out McFatties and a large cup of sugar. There were no food courts offering, fat, fatter or fattest options. There were no vending machines luring people to buy the best bad choice. Meat was lean and wild. Drink was out of a creek or a river. Fruit and vegetables were picked or dug. No gravy, no butter, no sugar, no hollandaise sauce, no icing, no, no, no, no, no. No cavewoman saying, "Does my ass look fat in my skimpy fur skirt?", "Does my club match my shoes", "What's for dessert?".

The food industry has done a fabulous job of making us fat! Each year they spend well over $400 million extolling the virtues of fast-food, high-sugar cereals, pop and candy. Once they have done a sufficient job of making Canadians obese, they come up with the low-fat scheme. Now they spend millions and millions of dollars telling us that what they sold us before has just been improved upon and is now low in fat. What they fail to tell us is in order for it to not taste like the packaging it came in, they have to fill it full of sugar. Now what happens when we consume too much sugar throughout the day, regardless of whether or not it has fat in it? If you can't burn it off, you store it—in fat cells. Period. Too much sugar equals excess calories, excess calories without exercise equals weight gain—even if you are eating low fat.

Does that mean that you shouldn't eat fat or does it mean you shouldn't eat low in fat? It means that nothing is easy! Most reputable nutrition books will recommend that no more than 30 per cent of your daily calories come from fat, regardless of whether they come in a box, a bowl, a can or a Ziploc bag. Now what does that mean? Take your plate and look at it, regardless of what you have on it. Does it look like more than 30 per cent of your plate is fat? This includes gravy, butter, sour cream, marbled steak, the oil you cooked your egg in, the peanut butter on your toast, the mayonnaise on your sandwich, the brownie for a snack and the cream in your coffee. Be honest with yourself.

It does not mean quit eating fat. It means get educated. Find out what foods have fat in them and how much. If you really want to get smart, look at how much saturated fat is in food because that is your dangerous fat. Now decide for yourself if the brownie is more important or the butter on your toast. Perhaps I'll give up the butter and sour cream on my potato in order to have steak instead of chicken. Maybe I'll have a two-egg omelet for breakfast but I'll eliminate one yolk. Maybe I'll switch from cream in my coffee to 2% milk. Switch from whole milk to 2%, then maybe even to 1% or skim. Maybe instead of eating that whole tub of Rolo ice-cream, I'll go to Dairy Queen and have one of their small, ice-milk cones. No cold turkey. No, "You can't have". No dying of taste malnourishment. No denying. No straight jackets or anti-depressants. Small choices, big changes. Fill the jug one drop at a time.

Eating late at night.

Have you ever noticed when you say the word *diet* you dream about food. You wake up in the middle of the night listening to Mr. Twinkie singing *Ding Dong the Low Fat Witch is Dead*. You get up, head to the big, white beast breathing rhythmically in the night waiting for your arrival at its doors. As you arrive, scratching your butt and yawning, you open the door to see an oasis of gifts begging you to sit down and open each and every one. Before you know it the chocolate cake from dinner that you were just dreaming was a hat, is but a pile of crumbs in your Joe Boxer lap. Now what happens? Do I vomit or do I go to bed? Vomiting takes too much energy and might really wake you up so you just go back to bed. Now what happens to all those calories you just consumed? The same thing that happened to the bowl of popcorn riddled with M & M's you ate last night at 9 p.m. while watching *Desperate Housewives*. Nothing! There is nothing for them to do but skip merrily down the bloodstream and knock on the closest fat cell door asking for a warm place to curl up and sleep—along with all the other happy fat that was stored from the night before. The women I spoke to found this to be their worst and most common food habit. Eating at night, after dinner, while watching television, too exhausted to make a conscious decision to put the food away. You had a long, hard, stressful day and you deserve this tub of ice-cream, damn it. Problem is you also deserve the consequences. A few moments in the mouth and an eternity on the butt.

Food was designed to be eaten in order to be burned as fuel in order to survive. When we consume vast quantities of calories at the time of day when we do the least amount of activity, those calories cannot be utilized, therefore they get stored in fat cells, regardless of whether they have any fat in them.

Portion control.

Yeah baby, super size me, then super size my butt too! Over the years, the portion sizes served in restaurants and sold in stores has increased dramatically. What used to be a six ounce steak, a medium baked potato, and seasonal vegetables is now a small cow, a bag of potatoes, and screw those seasonal veggies, throw in a loaf of bread and a block of butter, would yuh? What about seconds? What is that all about? Keep in mind that food was designed to be eaten in order to be burned as fuel in order to survive. Now ask yourself—with the amount I am eating, am I planning on surviving a famine?

Talking with so many women about their food habits has made me realize how much more food we eat, than our bodies require. Take a look at holiday dinners as an example. First off we wake up in the morning vowing not to eat until dinner so there will be more room in our stomach, therefore we can eat more. (What about the whole breakfast, metabolism, blood sugar levels blah, blah, blah—who cares, it's turkey!) Next we sip on alcoholic beverages throughout the afternoon to stave off those familiar waves of nausea and light headedness. (What about that whole blood sugar, insulin, fat cell, gate keeper blah, blah, blah—who cares, it's turkey!) Next we make sure to wear expandable clothing! Supper is served and by now a wooly mammoth, seeping snot would taste great. You load up your plate with turkey, gravy, mashed potatoes and butter, stuffing and gravy, carrots, peas, brussels sprouts, but only one because they are gross, sweet potatoes and a bun with butter to sop up the dregs. This first plate only takes 10 minutes to consume because you are so damn hungry! You start on seconds before the brain and the gut have had a chance to chit chat and say, "Dear God I'm full!" The second plate isn't nearly as full because you are watching your waist these days. Just a bit more turkey, mashed potatoes and stuffing with gravy. By the time the second plate is finished, the brain and the gut have had a chance to communicate and the stomach says, "You'll just never learn will you?". So what do you do? Go sit down for a while and let supper digest before dessert!

Sound familiar? Sadly it is pretty accurate. Now let's talk about other food occasions. Take buffet dinners—this is an overeating craze waiting to happen. You pay $12.95 for a breakfast buffet and you're going to damn well eat your $12.95 worth of food. We were in Las Vegas this past year and got to witness a buffet "American" style in one of the most decadent cities in the U.S. People eating three and four plates of food because they paid for it and it is instantly available and loaded with fat, which tastes so damn good. Meanwhile the poor salad section wilts like the short kid who is always picked last for the basketball game. What about super size me? Not quite enough fat and calories in a regular size order of processed potatoes fried in saturated fat so let's up the consequences a bit. What about big-gulp Slurpees, enormous buckets of theatre popcorn, colossal size Mr. Big chocolate bars, huge Dairy Queen Blizzards, three patty hamburgers, foot-long hot dogs, giant to-go mugs of coffee, 100 item buffets, and endless fries? I can honestly say I have never seen a super size me salad offer, and if you did, it would come with the super size salad dressing loaded with saturated fat and sugar. Don't get depressed, get educated.

Although the number of calories that should be consumed at any one sitting varies dramatically from person to person, we all have the potential to overeat. The fitter you are and the more active you are, the more muscle mass you will have on your frame and that translates into more calories that can be consumed at any given sitting. Here are some suggestions to help you think about and control your portion sizes.

- Avoid eating in front of the television or when you are in a hurry. Sit down at a table while you eat your food. This will help you to pay attention to how much you are consuming. Many times, the quantity of food that is consumed while watching television is simply because you are not paying attention to what is going in your mouth.
- Eat slowly so that your brain and your stomach have a chance to communicate. The faster you eat, the more you tend to eat before you realize you have eaten too much and are uncomfortably full. This is what often happens during holiday meals.

- Try to eat meals and snacks at regular intervals so that you don't get to the point that you are starving. This is when people tend to overeat.
- Pay close attention to serving sizes. When reading labels keep in mind that a serving size does not necessarily mean the whole can or the whole box. A can of soup is a good example. You may look at the label and think that it is a good choice but you may not realize that the label only refers to one-half or one-third of the can.
- Serve your meals on a smaller plate. This will make you feel like your plate is still full but it will help to cut down on the actual amount you are eating.
- If you are going to indulge in a high fat, high sugar snack, read the label and measure out one serving size. At least you will know exactly what you are consuming—then enjoy it.

"My worst food habit is eating way too much and way too often. I enjoy eating too much, I would rather be a sex addict!"

Interview Client #51

What about just not eating?

According to the video, *A Matter of Fat*, there are well over eight million obese people in Canada right now and that number is doubling every seven years. Why are we becoming such an obese society when the diet industry is the richest it has ever been? Billions and billions of dollars are spent on diet products in North America each year and we are the fattest we have ever been. It starts with not eating and ends with how much of what we are eating.

Every time a woman purchases another diet book or signs a

contract with another diet agency or buys another bottle of diet pills, she signs up for another version of the same stop-eating theory. If you just stop eating, you should be able to lose weight. Right? Wrong!

Each and every time we drastically reduce our caloric intake we provide a famine environment in our body. This famine environment is recognized by the brain and once again the brain tells the whole body to shut down in order to burn very few calories—very slowly. It is the only way it can make them last. The body will continue to do this for as long as you continue to starve it. Starving doesn't have to mean an anorexic diet. It is simply less calories than the body requires to survive in a 24-hour period, at rest. Finally after three months you reach your *goal* weight, wherever the hell that came from, and in the horizon you see the herd of cattle slowly approaching! You do well for the first week of maintenance and then decide you deserve to celebrate your success with dinner out. You start with a lovely order of roasted garlic and brie, which is in fact more calories than you have been consuming all day for the past three months. You settle on a pesto pasta for dinner thinking it is a healthy choice regardless of the fact the calorie content is equal to three days of your current caloric intake. You top this off with a glass of wine and a coffee drink with your low fat crème brulee. After dinner you realize what you have been missing for the past three months but vow to only celebrate your continued willpower on the weekends. Except for Melinda's birthday, Thanksgiving, the staff luncheon out, your birthday, and 43 pounds later you're four pounds heavier than you were when you started the last diet.

What is the problem here? The problem is you're consuming too many calories for a suppressed metabolism to deal with. Each and every time you go on a calorie restricted diet you commit metabolic sabotage. Each and every time you start to eat normally you are eating with a suppressed metabolism. Do this five times each year and each year you suppress your metabolism five times. Problem is it doesn't bounce back like your stomach after liposuction or your boobs after a boob job. Over time, it stays depressed and it will stay depressed until you begin to treat it the way it was meant to be treated. Nutritious food, throughout the day, in manageable amounts, along with activity. Simple! Like Nike says, "Just Do It".

What is in a pound anyway?

There are 3,500 calories in one pound of fat. There are four calories in one gram of protein and four calories in one gram of carbohydrates. There are nine calories in one gram of fat and seven calories in one gram of alcohol. In order to get rid of one pound of fat, not just one pound but one pound of fat, you must burn off 3,500 calories of stored body fat. Big difference between losing one pound of fat and losing one pound. Now the best way to burn off one pound of stored body fat is to get up and move. If you walked off 500 calories per day it would take you seven days to lose a pound of fat, if your diet didn't change. Imagine you would like to lose 50 pounds. Fifty pounds, times 3,500 calories, is 175,000 calories that need to be eliminated from your body through sensible eating and exercise. Simple changes such as eating several smaller meals throughout the day, decreasing your portion sizes, and exercising and you have a perfect environment for fat loss. No gimmicks, no contracts, no meetings, no measuring tapes, no hand-holding and weight loss prayers—just hard work.

Reading labels.

This can be a bit tricky and a little overwhelming so we are going to keep it very simple. Start reading what is in the food you are eating. There are so many ingredients that are hidden in food that we don't recognize as sugars or salts or fats. Let's start by saying the RDA advises a maximum of 40 grams of sugar per day. There are four grams of sugar in one teaspoon, that equals a maximum RDA of 10 teaspoons of sugar per day. Now go grab some of your boxes and look at how much sugar is listed in one serving and then take a look at how big a serving is.

Sugar can be disguised as glucose, sucrose, maltose, fructose, maple syrup, honey, molasses, dextrose, sorbitol, turbinado, amazake, carob powder, corn syrup and high fructose corn syrup to name a few. One of the most interesting foods to check the sugar content of is cereal. Take a cereal such as Raisin Bran, which is toted as a healthy cereal because of the bran, and notice the grams of sugar per serving are 16 grams. That is 40 per cent of your daily sugar requirement in one cup of cereal and your day is just beginning. Now take an item such as a piece of chocolate cake which contains 15 teaspoons of sugar or one-eighth of a quart of ice-cream which contains 23 teaspoons of sugar and you can see how easy it is to over-consume sugar. Remember that too much sugar in your diet gets stored in the fat cells, if it's not burned off.

How about fat? The advertising world got insidiously sneaky when they figured out how to hide the fat content of food, even though it has to be listed on the label. Grab a label and take a peek, preferably a salad dressing. When you read the label and you see there are only three grams of fat, you think—good choice. Now look at the serving size and the total calories. Serving size is one tablespoon. Who only puts one tablespoon of dressing on their salad? Total calories per serving is 50. If you do the math, that means your one tablespoon

of dressing is 54 per cent fat! That is not cool. In order to figure out what per cent of your calories are coming from fat,
simply take the fat grams—in this case three—multiply it by
nine, because there are nine calories in each gram of fat, and
then divide that by the total calories. In this case it would be
27 divided by 50 which equals 54 per cent. It is just as important to do this calculation as it is to read the labels. Of course
there are no labels to bother with when eating foods in their
natural state, such as fruits and veggies!

The following is a label from a commercial spaghetti sauce.
I have included the basic information required for determining
fat, sodium and sugar contents. I have left out vitamin and
mineral content. As you will notice, this label is based on a
one-half cup serving. The first thing to determine is whether
or not the serving size is reasonable. When looking at the
calorie content keep in mind that it does not include adding
additional ingredients, such as hamburger, to the sauce.

Nutrition Facts - Spaghetti Sauce
Per 1/2 cup serving

Calories per serving	90
Fat	3 g
Saturated	.5 g
Trans	0 g
Sodium	560 mg
Carbohydrates	13 g
Sugars	8 g
Protein	2 g

To determine the percentage of calories that come from fat we need to perform our basic mathematical equation—x number of fat grams times nine calories per gram (remember there are nine calories in every gram of fat) divided by the calories per serving. In this case it would be three grams of fat times nine fat calories divided by 90 calories per serving for a fat content of 30 per cent. Next is sodium. The recommended daily intake of sodium for adults is 2,400mg per day or the equivalent of about one teaspoon of table salt. This product has 560mg of sodium per serving or about 23 per cent of your daily requirements. Last is carbohydrates and more specifically, sugar. Keeping in mind that a 2,000 calorie diet should consume no more than nine teaspoons of sugar and one teaspoon of sugar is approximately 4.5 grams, this one-half cup serving has almost two teaspoons of sugar!

Next is a label from a popular commercial cereal. Notice this label is based on a serving size of 25 biscuits which does not include milk.

Nutrition Facts - Cereal
Per 25 biscuits

Calories per serving	190
Fat	1 g
Saturated	0 g
Trans	0 g
Sodium	0 mg
Carbohydrates	45 g
Sugars	13 g
Protein	4 g

Starting with fat, one gram of fat times nine calories divided by 190 equals less than one per cent fat. I'd say that is a good choice, even better if you choose to use skim or 1% milk. Next is sodium. Zero milligrams is pretty self-explanatory. Next is sugar. Thirteen grams of sugar, before milk, equates to approximately 2.5-3 teaspoons of sugar. That is still a pretty good choice, especially if it is for a child and is combined with a low fat milk.

Although we did not touch on fibre with the previous label, let's take a look at fibre with this label. For an adult consuming approximately 2,000 calories per day, fibre intake should be approximately 25 grams. This cereal has a fibre content of five grams per serving and the spaghetti sauce has a fibre content of three grams per serving.

Now let's take a creamy cucumber dressing and really get a mouth full. The serving size for this dressing is one tablespoon. I've said it before and I'll say it again, "Who only puts one tablespoon of dressing on their salad?" If you're like me, you put enough dressing on to produce a lake underneath the lettuce. Each tablespoon has 50 calories and five grams of fat. Five grams of fat times nine fat calories divided by 50 calories is 90 per cent fat. Each tablespoon of this dressing that is put on your *low fat* salad is equal to 90 per cent fat.

Each tablespoon of dressing contains 200 mg of sodium or approximately eight per cent of your daily requirement. Last is the sugar content. This dressing only has one gram of sugar. When you get used to reading labels and understanding what is in food, you'll begin to recognize that many foods give up the sugar for the fat and vice versa. Sugar and fat are what give food flavor. If food is low in fat, it is very often high in sugar and when it is low in sugar it is very often high in fat. I have

Nutrition Facts - Salad Dressing
Per 1 Tbsp.

Calories per serving	50
Fat	5 g
Saturated	.5 g
Trans	0 g
Cholesterol	0 mg
Sodium	200 mg
Carbohydrates	1 g
Fibre	0 g
Sugars	1 g
Protein	0 g

found that the best salad dressings are the ones you make from scratch. That way you control both the fat and the sugar content.

The last example is one that tends to be near and dear to a lot of women's hearts. Ice-cream! This is a label from vanilla flavored ice-cream with cookie dough and chocolate chip pieces.

Start with portion size. One half-cup? Not a chance! One half-cup equals approximately 8.5 tablespoons. That is like putting two quarters in a slot machine, winning 100 quarters and then walking away. Let's say for argument sake that you manage to measure out one-half cup and you sit down and eat it slowly. Nine fat calories times nine calories divided by 170 equals 48 per cent fat. Each spoonful of this ice-cream is almost 50 per cent fat.

Nutrition Facts - Ice-cream

Per 1/2 cup serving

Calories per serving	170
Fat	9 g
Saturated	6 g
Trans	.4 g
Cholesterol	15 mg
Sodium	60 mg
Carbohydrates	23 g
Fibre	0 g
Sugars	18 g
Protein	1 g

Just to compound your misery, look at the saturated fat. Sixty-six per cent of that fat is saturated. That means when you eat it, it eventually looks like the marbled fat in a steak, in your system. Mmmmmmm. What about cholesterol and sodium? Not bad. How about sugar? Well, we know that ice-cream is one of those gifts in life that tastes like sweet velvet cream because it has both fat and sugar—but how much sugar? This particular ice-cream has 18 grams of sugar per serving or 3.5-4 teaspoons of sugar. Now let's be a bit more realistic about portion size. Take your cup or cup-and-a-half and double or triple those figures. You decide if it's worth it.

Take the time to pay attention to labels, they are like a scratch and win for your thighs. Low in fat, low in sugar, low in sodium—a winner! Don't let the marketing gurus trick you into believing that food is healthier than it is. It is up to *you* to start learning which foods are healthy choices and which ones are deceptively unhealthy. Start paying attention to sugar content and sodium content as well as fat content and overall calories. Don't get overwhelmed, it's not rocket science, it just takes a bit of recognizing and a lot of learning. Buy a food content book and a fat ruler and keep them in your purse. If you're not sure, pull out your fat ruler, line up the fat and the calories and voila—fat percentage. Now read the ingredient list. Look for the menacing sugar, sodium, chemicals and various fats disguised as words we can't pronounce.

Menu planning

It's 6 p.m., you've just left work and picked up the kids from soccer practice. You have nothing organized for dinner and you don't feel like going to the grocery store. By the time you get home and cook, it will be 7:30 p.m. You're tired and they are hungry. McDonald's, Wendy's, A&W or Kraft Dinner? One more night won't matter. But it will.

Are these the messages you want to send your children? I'm not organized. I don't feel like cooking. Fast food is a good alternative. Eating in the vehicle is quality time together. Cooking is a chore. Nutrition isn't important. Once a week isn't a big deal. Vegetables are overrated. Good things come in small boxes. The food is cheap. You're young, so it doesn't matter. It won't catch up to you. It's a treat.

If you have a busy, hectic life and health and nutrition are important to you and your family, then menu planning is not an option. When you are making dinner at night, start to think about what you are going to make for dinner the next night or make enough so there will be leftovers for tomorrow night.

Before you leave the house in the morning, take what you need out of the freezer. If you work close to a grocery store, pop out at lunch and pick up what you need for dinner. On the weekend organize your menu for the upcoming week and get the groceries you are going to require. If you have to do some prepping to make life easier, do it all on the same day. Cut the lettuce, wash it and spin it and stick it in a Tupperware bin. Cut all your veggies up and place them in baggies or plastic containers. Make a large container of salad dressing. Bake enough cookies for two weeks and freeze them. Double your spaghetti or chili recipe and freeze half of it. Make sure you have enough breakfast, lunch and snack items on hand. Not only will this help with your weight loss success but it will make a huge difference in your wallet at the end of the month.

If you really dislike cooking, educate yourself about healthy pre-packaged choices such as perogies, healthy canned soups, healthy pasta sauce options, pre-made salads, frozen dinners. It is obviously much more expensive to eat this way but if you're not going to cook, then plan your menu with these options in mind. At the very least try to throw together a salad to go along with your perogies or canned soups. It takes nothing to make a salad if you have pre-washed the lettuce and pre-cut all the veggies. Don't let menu planning be an option.

Grazing

Grazing means taking your 1,500 or 1,800 calories per day and spreading them out over five or six snacks rather than over three meals. Imagine you are eating 1,200 calories per day. You have your piece of toast and an apple for breakfast, your pre-packaged salad and Wasa bread for lunch. By the time you get home you are ravenous. All you've eaten today is less than 500 calories which means you still have over 700 calories left to go. Now think about the time of day that you are likely to consume the greatest number of calories and you can see that it is going to be an excellent way to gain weight. Seven hundred calories at one sitting is too much for someone who is trying to lose weight, has a sedentary job and doesn't do anything at night. Try taking those 1,200 calories and break them down into six, 200 calorie snacks or four, 300 calorie snacks. Not only will you stabilize your blood sugar which in turn stabilizes your moods and your ability to focus, but you won't feel hungry. If you are constantly feeding your metabolism a little bit all day long, it will slowly learn to burn more efficiently.

Routine

It is important to establish routine in your weight management quest. If you know exactly what is expected of you on any given day, it takes the guess work out of an already complicated issue. Eat breakfast at the same time each morning. Have a selection of three or four simple breakfasts and leave it at that. Get up early enough to pack your lunch and organize your thoughts for dinner. Establish the best time of day for you to exercise and don't waver from that schedule unless there is an emergency. If it is a morning walk that works best for you, ensure that your shoes and clothes are laid out and ready for you. If you are better at exercising after work, make sure you have your gym bag packed and in the car. Try to eat dinner within the same time frame each night and ensure you have leftovers for tomorrow's lunch. After dinner, go for a walk, sit down and read or organize your food and clothes for tomorrow. Make Monday to Friday a work week at home, just like it is for work. On the weekend, maintain a schedule but a loose schedule. Take one day to get some sort of exercise, do your grocery shopping for the week, wash, chop and store your veggies, make some soup, stew or sauces for the freezer, and organize the family to help you do the laundry and housework so that it is done for the upcoming week. Relax and enjoy your successes.

The less guess work you have in your hectic work week, the greater the chance of success with your eating, exercise and weight loss/weight management program. Imagine if you just flew by the seat of your pants every day, the chances of making poor food choices increases, the chances of you getting your exercise decreases and the chances of frustration, stress and anxiety are inevitable.

Spot reduction

Regardless of what *The South Beach Diet* tells you, you cannot will pounds away from certain areas of your body. If that were the case, I would will some fat from my head to my boobs and my calves and I would will my hair straight. *The South Beach Diet* claims that the majority of the weight you lose in the first two weeks of the diet will be from your waistline. When you think logically about this statement, you will realize if the majority of the weight you have to lose is from your waistline, that is likely where you are going to notice the loss.

The body is a clever combination of connective tissue and nerve endings designed to survive regardless of the irrational things our mind tells it to do. Jane Fonda told us to 'Go for the burn', Suzanne Sommers told us, 'We must, we must, we must increase our bust', fitness gurus led us to believe that 500 sit-ups a day would give us a washboard abdomen, and websites outline what to do to have a body like your favorite celebrity. Well, I am here to tell you that all these statements are, at best, being economical with the truth. Sure you can go for the burn but your likely going to end up with an injury. The only way to increase your bust size is by getting fat, pregnant or purchasing a new set of perky breast implants. Doing 500 sit-ups per day is going to give you a tight abdomen but you'll never see it if you don't get rid of the fat lying on top of it. The only way you will have a body like your favorite celebrity is if you were built like them in the first place.

There is no such thing as spot reduction. There is, however, such a thing as spot toning. If you want flat abs, do lots of core strengthening exercises. If you want bigger biceps, do lots of bicep curls. If you want a butt like a dancer, do lots of squats and lunges. If you want to tone those hammocks hanging off the back of your arms, do lots of triceps exercises. I say this emphatically but with a disclaimer. As long as you continue to eat the same way and don't include activities that will burn stored fat, the only person that will appreciate those newly-toned muscles is you, along with those happy fat cells that are concealing the muscle.

Contrary to popular belief, we all have abs, we all have toned thighs and we all have a cute butt, it's just that some of our body parts are hidden beneath a layer of fat that is a little bit thicker than other people's layer of fat. Some people's layer of fat is dimply and some people's layer of fat is squishy. Some people carry their layer of fat on their hips and butt and some people carry their layer of fat around their waistline and their back. Some people store fat easily and some people store fat quickly. Regardless of our genetic fat-blueprint, underneath, we all have the same muscles, in the same places, responsible for the same thing and it does not matter how much we work them, without proper nutrition, it won't change the layer of fat that is keeping them warm. Along with perky breasts heading south, one of the bodies' cruel jokes is—where you gain weight first, is usually the last place it comes off. Back to spot reducing. If you gain weight around your waist when you put on weight, are sit-ups going to get rid of it? No. If you have been on a diet for three months and still have five nasty pounds left and they are all around your waist, are sit-ups going to get rid of them? No. If you go off your diet and go back to your old eating habits, are you going to gain weight around your waist? Yes. It is what it is. Weight on, wait off. You can't change how your body stores fat, you can only recognize it, understand it, and work within it. If it is that important to you and you are willing to work hard enough, it will only be a matter of time until you achieve the results you desire. The only true method of spot reduction is called liposuction.

Body Mass Index

Body mass index is a popular tool used to gauge whether or not a person is overweight (if you don't already know). BMI is calculated by dividing a person's weight (in kilograms) by his/her height (in meters, squared).   This number represents your body weight category.

This is a great starting point for men and women who are sick of living their lives by the scale. The chart gives people a bit more information, in terms of their relative risk category, although most overweight people don't need to be told this. For those people who have no idea where to start, this is a great tool although the chart does not work well for people who are naturally lean or are overly muscular.

If you have not calculated your body mass index before, simply plug your height and weight into the following chart to determine your BMI. Next, take your waist measurement and voila, you have an excellent start point for your weight loss and lifestyle modification program.

BMI range	Category	Waist size less than or equal to 40" for men - 35" for women.	Waist size greater than 40" for men - 35" for women.
18.5 or less	Underweight		
18.5 - 24.9	Normal		
25.0 - 29.9	Overweight	Increased	High
30.0 - 34.9	Obese	High	Very high
35.0 - 39.9	Obese	Very high	Very high
40 or greater	Extremely obese	Extremely high	Extremely high

BMI Height (in)	19	20	21	22	23	24	25	26	27	28	29	30	35	40
				weight in pounds										
63	107	113	118	124	130	135	141	146	152	158	163	169	197	225
64	110	116	122	128	134	140	145	151	157	163	169	174	204	232
65	114	120	126	132	138	144	150	156	162	168	174	180	210	240
66	118	124	130	136	142	148	155	161	167	173	179	186	216	247
67	121	127	134	140	146	153	159	166	172	178	185	191	223	255
68	125	131	138	144	151	158	164	171	177	184	190	197	230	262
69	128	135	142	149	155	162	169	176	182	189	196	203	236	270
70	132	139	146	153	160	167	174	181	188	195	202	207	243	278
71	136	143	150	15	165	172	179	186	193	200	208	215	250	286
72	140	147	154	162	169	177	184	191	199	206	213	221	258	294

Glycemic Index

The glycemic index is a scale that has been around for over 20 years. It ranks carbohydrate-rich foods by how much they raise blood sugar or blood-glucose levels. When we eat carbohydrate-rich foods, the sugar from the food (glucose) breaks down during digestion and is used for energy. It is our simplest form of energy. Once the food is broken down and glucose is produced, the level of glucose in a person's system rises. It is the speed which the glucose level rises that is referred to as the 'glycemic response'. This response is influenced by such things as quantity of food, type of food and the way food is cooked. The less food is cooked, the lower the glycemic response.

This is an important factor to consider since choosing foods with a low glycemic response may help to control blood glucose levels, control your appetite, lower your risk of heart disease and Type II diabetes and control cholesterol levels. This is why so many diets have been based on the low carbohydrate concept. What many diets fail to consider are low GI (glycemic index) carbs vs. high GI carbs. Low GI carbs are essential to a healthy diet and can be combined with medium GI carbs to slow down the glycemic response. A GI of 55 or less ranks as low, a GI of 56-69 is ranked as medium, a GI of 70 or more ranks as high.

Glucose levels in the bloodstream are what stimulate the pancreas to secrete insulin. Insulin is a hormone which moves glucose from the bloodstream into the muscles and the fat cells. The more glucose, the more insulin, the more storing. The lower the GI rating of food, the less glucose that is produced, the less insulin, the less fat storing.

Some basic guidelines to follow in order to lower your glycemic index on a daily basis include limiting the amount of processed food and refined starchy food. Eat whole grains, legumes and lentils. Combine low and medium GI foods. Decrease the cooking time of foods and try to eat vegetables in as close to their natural state as possible. Limit portion sizes; the bigger the portion, the more it will increase your blood glucose level, regardless of its GI ranking. Lastly, familiarize yourself with the GI ranking of food. Go to the search engine Google and type—*Glycemic Index Chart.* Print off a copy and keep it handy in the kitchen for when you are preparing meals as well as a copy in your purse for when you are shopping. This will make it very easy to ensure you make appropriate GI choices.

But exercise makes me sweat!

I won't spend much time on exercise because I have included a whole chapter on it but let's just say that calories that go in have to get out somehow and the only way is to get up and get moving. The less active we are, the happier our fat cells are going to be. Losing weight has little to do with not eating and a whole lot to do with getting up and moving. Figure out what activity you are going to include in your life, for life.

5

THE DIET REVIEW

I decided if I was to understand the nature of habitual dieting, I needed to understand the characteristics of the game. In order to understand that, I had to familiarize myself with the most common games that women participated in. I have reviewed 10 of the most popular diets as of January, 2007. I tried to remain open-minded, like a juror on a media-crazed murder case. Sometimes that was more difficult than the diet I was reviewing.

The Atkins Diet—This diet was developed in 1972 by Dr. Atkins. It remains as controversial as it is challenging. I had to keep asking myself, "How could anyone subscribe to a diet that instructs you to remove fruits and vegetables and to eat as much cream, cheese, bacon, eggs and other saturated fats as you like"? It doesn't promote or establish portion sizes or encourage exercise or lifestyle management strategies. No wonder it is so popular!

The premise of this diet is that we have become a carbohydrate-crazed society. Diets made up primarily of carbohydrates can cause insulin resistance and unstable blood sugar levels. Carbohydrate-rich diets tend to promote the burning of stored carbohydrates as our main form of energy rather than fats. Dr. Atkins designed this diet to train our bodies to utilize fats for energy, thereby burning more stored fat and less stored carbohydrates. I like this concept since it is obvious that we all store considerably more fat than we do carbohydrates, but the appeal of the diet is limited to this concept. It made me question the plan when Dr. Atkins was considered obese and suffering from heart disease and hypertension at the time of his death. It is claimed that these factors were a result of a medical condition and that he died of a head injury sustained in a fall.

The diet itself is a four-phase game. The first phase, called the *Induction Phase*, lasts two weeks, although some reviews state that you can stay on this phase for as long as you are able to manage. During this stage, the willing participant reduces their carbohydrate intake to 20 grams or less per day. That is about enough carbohydrates to complete 14 sit-ups or the drive to drop off the kids at school, but not back. No fruit, very few vegetables, no sweets, no refined foods, no juice, no pasta, no rice, no, no, no, no, no—but go for it with the cream cheese, New York steak and brie. The reward for this punishment is to switch the body from sugar-burning mode to fat-burning mode. During this restriction phase, the body produces ketones from fat which are then used as our fuel source instead of carbohydrates or glucose. Go directly to diet jail. Do not pass "GO", do not collect $200.

In diet jail you will likely receive headaches, low energy, fatigue and an inability to concentrate. This may be due to a lack of brain food which comes from carbohydrates. On the bright side, meal time will be a protein and fat buffet with none of that salad crap.

Phase two of this game is called the *Ongoing Weight Loss Phase*. Assuming you have lost weight eating steak and cheese for each meal, and are still coherent enough to progress to phase two, you get to increase your carbohydrate consumption from 20 grams per day to 40-50 grams per day. In other words, from three cups of loosely packed lettuce to six cups of loosely packed lettuce. Throughout this phase you are encouraged to monitor how your body is reacting to the diet. Giggle. Pretty sure I know how the body is reacting and it's not cute. Husband and kids aren't enjoying you very much and you don't smell all that great. Butter without the potato is getting boring. Steak without potatoes is getting boring. Brie without crackers is getting boring. Peanut butter without bread or chocolate chips is getting boring. Cheese without the baguette is getting boring. A hotdog without the bun is getting boring. A hamburger without the ketchup, lettuce, tomatoes, pickles, and onions on a toasted sesame seed bun, just isn't a hamburger.

Phase three is the *Pre-Maintenance Phase* and it begins when the participant is five to 10 pounds away from their goal weight—I couldn't quite figure out how that was established. Carbohydrates are increased again, this time to a level called the "critical carbohydrate level". This is the level where, if you don't get to eat them soon, you're going to dig Dr. Atkins up just so you can have a little chat with him. In this phase, weight loss is slowed down in preparation for the final phase. Less than one pound of weight per week is to be lost at the end of this phase. Your critical carbohydrate level is established while in phase two and is determined by how many carbohydrates you can eat while still losing weight. Apparently you need a physiology-carbohydrate degree for this game.

The final phase is called the *Maintenance Diet*. This phase is aimed at keeping the dieter at their "target" weight, for life. The dieter will have to keep their carbohydrate intake restricted to a level that will maintain their weight.

Although I can't imagine playing this game for life, I believe it may have a place in certain situations and it does have a couple of merits. First off, it may be a good option for people who suffer from hypoglycemia, are severely insulin resistant or are carbohydrate junkies.

A lot of foods are allowed on this diet that typically aren't included in traditional diets which makes it a bit more liberal. I did question the effect this diet may have on people with high cholesterol and heart disease but could not find any long term studies that showed any significant results. Lastly, any diet that promotes supplementing with multivitamins to make up for what you are missing because of food restriction, is a concern. Of the 74 reviews that I read, 20 per cent gave the diet a 5/5, 24 per cent gave it a 4/5, 12 per cent gave it a 3/5, 16 per cent gave it a 2/5 and 28 per cent gave it a 1/5.

Should you stay away from this diet? Not necessarily. If you have done your homework and understand the diet inside and out and it makes sense to you, perhaps you should try it. If you think you can sustain this program for life, perhaps it is right for you. If you are a carbohydrate-crazed, hypoglycemic, insulin-resistant, junk-food junkie, perhaps this is a good alternative. But, if you love fruits and veggies, you are a vegetarian or you're Italian, don't bother because by the end of week one you will want to eat the unsweetened baking chocolate hiding in the cupboard from five years ago. Remember that the key to a good nutrition and weight loss plan is one that fits your lifestyle, for life.

Body For Life—This game was developed by former competitive body builder, Bill Phillips, which in itself should scare you. He is also the founder of EAS nutritional supplements, therefore any supplements that are recommended for this game likely won't come in "no-name" brand packaging. The principles outlined in Mr. Phillips' program are very popular in the bodybuilding realm but have been wrapped up in a consumer-friendly package so that it appeals to the general public. When I worked in the fitness industry, I watched a lot of gym members play this game. Very few with much success because of the level of exercise required. Those who were successful were gym rats that already spent considerable time in the gym. I was quite interested in this particular diet because I watched so many people attempt it when it was "the" next great diet.

The rules to this game are simple: diet, exercise, portion control, grazing, increased protein and lots of water. It starts out sounding viable until you read the fine print, starting with exercise. Anyone that exercises as much as this program prescribes is going to lose weight regardless of what they eat. If you are not a gym rat and have never done any weight lifting you will probably quit this diet after the first lower body workout because your legs will be so sore you won't be able to get off the toilet. If going to the bathroom or walking are not a necessity in your life, then this may be a useful game to play. You work out six days a week, rotating between lower body and upper body workouts and aerobic workouts. Mr. Phillips has a prescription of exercises, sets, reps, tempo, duration, and intensity. If you don't know the difference between a set and a rep or a bicep and a deltoid, you may need to take along your exercise physiology book, sold by EAS products. It's called *Body for Life* but chances of you doing this workout regime for life are slim. Beware of the before-and-after pictures, they are meant to sell you on the concept and are a bit optimistic for the average person.

The diet promotes an increase in low fat proteins and a decrease in refined carbohydrates, smaller portion sizes, grazing and lots of water. On the seventh day, you are free to eat whatever you like. I like all of these concepts except the "get out of jail free" day. When I was reading reviews from people who had tried this diet, many of them said that the *free* day was the best part of the program because they could eat however much of whatever they wanted. This could end up being a bit counterproductive if you struggle with food addictions. The program recommends six small meals spaced approximately three hours apart with portion sizes resembling your fist. This is good advice, if you are super-organized, can limit your food intake to fist-size portions, don't mind dictating your day by an egg timer and aren't always eating on the run. I had a hard time finding reviews from people who had participated in the *Body for Life* program but of the 21 that I did find, 71 per cent gave it a 5/5, 24 per cent gave it a 4/4 and 5 per cent gave it 2/5.

Should you play this game? If you love the gym, don't eat out much, are super-organized and extremely committed, this may be a good option for you. If you hate weight training, going to the gym, grocery shopping and you eat on the fly, don't waste your money on the book or your time reading the book because it won't work for you. Coming from a fitness perspective, I can see how this program could be very successful for a small portion of the population. I like some of the rules that Mr. Phillips outlines in his game, especially exercising, but I question most people's ability to make the appropriate changes for life. It is called *Body for Life* but the chances of you being able to do it for life are not great. Remember that the key to a good nutrition and weight loss plan is one that fits your lifestyle, for life.

L.A. Weight Loss—I was really looking forward to learning the rules to this game because it is so heavily promoted in the media right now. Too bad I was disappointed. Same thing, different spin. Buy our stuff. Sign here. No information over the phone. Questionably qualified "weight loss counselors". Two steps forward, one step back. Three phases. Thanks to La La Weight Loss, I lost 48 pounds in two weeks. Blah, blah, blah.

L.A. Weight Loss has been around since the late 80s and is a franchise operation so the quality of service and level of knowledge may vary from centre to centre. I found it very odd that information about the program would not be given over the phone. Although I understand why companies do this, I believe if you trust the product or service you are selling, you want to get the information out to as many people as possible, any way that you can. The same holds true for communicating with the counselors—in person only—which can be tough if you live in Aklavik.

Phase one is the weight loss phase. Professor Plum is assigned a caloric intake between 1,100 and 1,800 calories a day based on information acquired by the "counselor". After the professor reaches her goal weight—which again is a questionably acquired piece of data—she moves out of phase one and into phase two, the stabilization phase. This phase lasts six weeks.   The final phase of poor Professor Plum's diet is the maintenance phase. I wish just one company would use a more interesting word like preservation or perpetuation phase, it sounds a bit more naughty and fun. This final phase allows the good professor to "reintroduce" junk back into her diet.

Hmmmm, eliminate food, buy our expensive supplements and bars, sign our contracts—in blood, empty your wallet, exercise to our videos, chat—in person—with our "counselors", who are successful La La Weight Loss participants and have been trained in-house, show up several times per week—in person—to check in, live by a caloric intake assigned by non-registered professionals, pay up front, temporary routines. Take the information and decide for yourself.

On the flip side of the coin—and there are always two sides to a coin—for your hard earned dough, willing participants are given lists of appropriate foods to eat while eating out at popular restaurants. The diet allows alcohol, in moderation. A vegan plan is available and it does encourage exercise. There is a lot of one-to-one support, even if the counselors' education is questionable, and for many women, support is a big part of their weight loss success. Who to understand better than one who has gone through it? In general there doesn't seem to be anything glaringly valuable or potentially dangerous, other than the cost. I could not find a simple review site to establish how people were rating this program, I did however, find plenty of sites where people vented their displeasure with the program. If you wish to read testimonials, go to the Internet and search, *L.A. Weight Loss* Reviews. Should you play? If it seems like a viable nutrition and weight loss plan that will fit your lifestyle, for life.

Jenny Craig—Again I was curious about this program

because it has been around for so long and, of course, because Kirstie Ally has made it such a household name. I was pleasantly surprised—until I started to read the individual reviews. The program began in 1983 in Australia by a woman named— Jenny Craig. It opened operations in the United States in 1985 and now boasts over 600 centers in five countries. There are some definite benefits to this program, unfortunately they are outweighed by the company's product sales motivation.

Once again, the game is based on a three-tiered approach to weight loss, conveniently named, level one, two and three, for those of us who are verbally challenged. Level one teaches the participants how to eat the food they want, (that you have to buy from JC) but in smaller, more frequent portions. Level two teaches the participant how to increase their energy level by introducing exercise (convenient JC tapes recommended for a fee) or activity into their day. The third and final level teaches the participant how to build more balance into their lives, (JC motivational tapes recommended for a fee) in order to maintain their weight.

There are three different plans available, *The Jenny TuneUp*, *Jenny OnTrack* and the *Jenny Rewards*. I couldn't tell if these were exciting new names for the *10 pounds for $10 Plan*, the *Gold Plan* and the *Platinum Plan* or something completely different. I did figure out that each one is progressively more expensive than the previous and that the *Platinum Program* means you are a client for life. Lucky you. *The Jenny TuneUp* is designed for participants who have 15 pounds or less to lose. *Jenny OnTrack* offers the basic weight loss components plus weekly consultations with a weight-loss, JC-trinket salesperson. *The Jenny Rewards* adds a weight maintenance component, unlimited comeback privileges and gives the participant various discounts and rebates, (remember the more you spend, the more you save). Along with the three levels and the three plans, the program includes three elements that are crucial to weight loss. This part I liked.

The first element is food. The idea is to teach the participant about portion control, variety, and avoiding food group eliminations and the pitfalls of eating out. The second element is the body. The program promotes and encourages activity. Hallelujah. A weight-loss, JC-trinket salesperson helps the participant recognize barriers to being physically active—but don't take up too much of her valuable merchandise-selling time. The third element is the mind.

This is when the JC Host inspires the participant to surround herself with positive people and affirmations, in order to ensure success.

Okay, now that we have the basic concepts—how beneficial is the program? Ignoring my gentle sarcasm, I actually did find some useful aspects to this program. I liked the fact that you can get most of the information you want, either over the phone or on-line, except for hard costs. I found the 24/7 support system impressive. I loved the fact that activity is very strongly encouraged and that they define it as activity and not necessarily exercise. The fact that the menu plans are nutritionally balanced according to the USDA Food Guide and the U.S. Dietary Guidelines gives the program credibility. The fact that you can participate in this program both on-site or on-line opens it up to anyone, anywhere. *Jenny Craig* is advised by a medical advisory board including certified professionals in medicine, psychology and nutrition. There are no "bad" foods and no food groups are eliminated. Clients supplement their science-project meals with fruits and veggies. Lastly, moderation, not elimination, is strongly encouraged.

Now the flip side of the coin. JC's program is based on its pre-packaged, arrive in a box, just-add-water meals that will run you up to $100 per week. This may work well for someone who is very overweight and has a hard time thinking for themself or someone who hates to cook or is a single person. Once you add in the whole, 'I love to cook', 'I have a family', 'I can't afford it', 'Why don't I just buy frozen diet meals from the grocery store' concept—the program starts to tremble. I had a very difficult time finding individual reviews that praised the flavor of the individually served science-projects, but I figure if you are used to eating whatever you want, nothing on a diet is going to excite you. Next, the support staff. Since these are individually owned JC centers, the quality of the staff is going to vary. Regardless, it is important for participants to realize that these are not trained nutritionists, dieticians or psychologists. These are nice people, in need of a job, that are expected to sell, sell, sell. This was the part of the program that I found the most disappointing. All of the reviews that I read focused on the pressure to buy JC products and this held true for both the positive and the negative reviews.

So what is the verdict? If you have lots of dough, flavor isn't a big issue, you don't mind your groceries arriving by FedEx and you don't like to cook, this may be a great option. If you believe that weight loss is about changing your relationship with food and exercise and not about buying products, chances are this is not going to suit your needs. Should you play? Perhaps. There seems to be a lot of people who have lost weight on this program but whether or not they kept it off is another question. Of the 55 reviews that I read, 24 per cent gave the diet a 5/5, 31 per cent gave it 4/5, 11 per cent gave it a 3/5, 18 per cent gave it a 2/5 and 16 per cent gave it a 1/5.

Can you do it for life? If you're rich. Does JC want you to

do it for life? Yes and no. The company wants to eventually wean you off their food and back onto "normal" food but they also strongly recommend the participants up-sell to the lifetime program, in case the need ever arises.

Weight Watchers—I kept my fingers crossed when researching this program because I had so many clients who had such great success with the program. I had referred a lot of people to Weight Watchers, but I really only understood the basic principles and hadn't done any deep scratching to learn the real 'ins' and 'outs' of the program. What I learned helped to confirm this is a viable program.

Weight Watchers was founded by Jean Nidetch in the early 60s in the living room of her New York home. Now, millions of men and women around the world, have successfully participated in the program. Next to *E-diets*, *Weight Watchers* appears to be the top choice of critics, for a successful weight loss program. The program encourages a sensible diet consisting of healthy, ordinary foods, exercise and a positive attitude. No pre-packaged foods and no food is off limits. It is also very flexible, which makes it easy to follow, and the cost is very reasonable, less than $75 per month, which compared to other commercial weight loss programs, is cheap. In-person group meetings and weigh-ins are the cornerstone of the *Weight Watchers* diet plan and statistics have shown that those who participate in the support group component have better weight loss and weight management success. The food plan requires strict calorie control, but it does not require the purchase of pre-packaged food. It encourages activity, through a simple "points spender", awarding members points based on activity.

Currently, *Weight Watchers* is based on two plans. The *Flex Plan*, which is the cornerstone of the original *Weight*

Watchers program. This plan promotes healthy eating and calorie counting through a point system. Food is assigned a point value based on its fat, fibre and calorie content. In turn, the participant is assigned a daily point range based on their gender, height and weight. *Weight Watchers* also provides recipes with points already calculated, points for various restaurant foods and points for luxuries such as alcohol and desserts. Some restaurants have begun to include *Weight Watchers* meals and there are many *Weight Watchers* recipe books available, with the points conveniently calculated. Although I am not a believer in height/weight statistics, I found it encouraging that *Weight Watchers* assigned a range, based on this information. The initial goal for *Weight Watchers'* clients is a weight loss of 5-10 per cent and an ultimate weight goal of a BMI less than 25. For those participants who are extremely overweight, an incremental goal of 10 per cent at a time is established. This makes an overwhelming goal seem much more manageable. Activity, not necessarily exercise, was a priority. Again, points were assigned for activity based on body weight, time and intensity. Simple activities such as taking the stairs, parking at the far end of a parking lot and taking a walk, were included. Through simple mathematics, participants could eat slightly more points if they took their 'points spent' into consideration.

The second plan is called the *Core Plan*. This is relatively new for *Weight Watchers* and is based on the original program but allows members to control their calories by focusing their eating on a core list of nutritious foods, but without the counting or the tracking. This works well for people who like a bit more freedom and don't require as much hand-holding. Foods on this list are all low in fat and calories and include foods from all of the food groups. *Core Plan* members have a self-monitoring method involving a "comfort zone" scale to assess hunger and fullness on an ongoing basis. These members don't necessarily use tracking methods to monitor calories in and out.

Weight Watchers provides useful tools such as a journal called the *Quik Trak System* for recording food choices, as well as a *Points Tracker* for recording activity. *Weight Watchers* also has an online program that includes progress charts, full restaurant and grocery browse charts, calculators for caloric expenditure information as well as hundreds of recipes and meal ideas. They have also made this information available in a program called, *On-the-Go*, for handheld devices. *Weight Watchers* online program also provides a science library of articles that detail research backing all of the plan's principles and philosophies. I read 67 reviews from various members who participated in the *Weight Watchers* program—48 per cent gave it a 5/5, 40 per cent gave it a 4/4, 6 per cent gave it a 3/5, 5 per cent gave it a 2/5 and 1 per cent gave it a 1/5.

Is this the right program for you? Again, it is a matter of researching and establishing whether or not this form of eating meets your lifestyle needs. If you are not motivated to look up and record foods, this probably won't work for you unless you are self-directed enough to follow the *Core Plan* program. If you do not like group meetings or the structure of weekly meetings, you probably won't last on this program. If you don't think you have the discipline to eat healthy food instead of processed food, regardless of whether or not you are sticking to your daily points allotment, this may not be the program for you. However, if you like to have structure, guidelines, group support, accountability meetings, and you like to chart and record your progress and set-backs this is probably a great program for you. I appreciate the fact there are no food group eliminations, the program is designed to make you accountable for your food choices, it promotes and encourages activity and exercise, provides a tremendous amount of information on food choices, menu planning, recipes and restaurant choices and basically takes the guess work out of food choices and options. I recognize the value of the points trackers and activity calculators that can be tucked away in your purse for instant access. Overall, I found this program to be very beneficial in re-training the way people think about food choices and portion sizes. I found that once people have established a mental picture of portion size, they rarely go back to their old way of thinking. As well, once they realize just how calorie dense "luxury" foods can be, they tend to find it easier to limit or eliminate these foods from their diet.

Overall, I think *Weight Watchers* is a great program. Generally speaking, the medical and professional reviews that I read tended to support this same thinking. I believe that *Weight Watchers* has the potential to continue helping millions of people around the world as long as they keep the program based on the original concept and don't buy into "new and improved" slick marketing concepts. Should you run out and join WW's? Only if you have done your research and believe this is a program that suits your life and you can include it in your life, for life.

The Slim-Fast Program—This diet managed to elicit either glowing or scathing reports, although admittedly I found considerably more glowing than scathing reports, much to my surprise. There were no phases, steps or contracts to this program just basic information along with *Slim-Fast* products. I was surprised to learn that, as recent as January 2007, the *Slim-Fast* meal-replacement program was rated as the second best weight loss program by consumer reports. According to www.bestweightlossprogram4me.com, there have been over 30 published clinical trials proving its effectiveness over the years. A clinical trial by The North American Association for the Study of Obesity found that people who used the *Slim-Fast* program, on and off for 10 years, were on an average 33 pounds lighter than a similar group who had not used *Slim-Fast*.

How does it work? Well, it is mind-numbingly easy, if you disregard the willpower portion of the program. Six small meals/snacks spread out throughout the day, three of which are meant to either be, or include, the *Slim-Fast* meal replacement products. You choose which meals or snacks are *Slim-Fast* and which are sensible, portion controlled meals. There is no calorie counting, carb counting, or points counting. *Slim-Fast* has over 100 products, many of which are available in the grocery store, are relatively affordable and are apparently quite palatable. I was surprised to learn that their website has registered dietitians available to answer questions and for doctors, whose patients are following the *Slim-Fast* plan, the website also provides medical guidelines. *Slim-Fast* encourages 30 minutes of daily activity.

On the flip side, there were several articles that questioned the overall daily caloric intake and the nutritional quality of the products. One woman referred to the diet as, Death by Milkshake. I can't help but wonder how anyone can live off meal replacements for the rest of their lives. It is obvious what will happen when they go back to eating normally. The program doesn't really teach portion control, proper food choices, food variety, or lifestyle changes. It appears to be more of a kick starter or a temporary weight loss plan, although according to their website, it has been shown to be effective for long-term weight management in published studies of one, two, four and five year's duration. Once again, I could not find a reliable site that showed reviews of people who had participated in the plan.

Finally, is this a viable weight loss program? Possibly. If your culinary desires are limited, you eat on the go a lot, you are single, and lead a relatively sedentary lifestyle. Could you live by this program for life? Probably not, but who knows, there are people all over the world that only eat rice!

The South Beach Diet—Alakabam! With a wave of the hand, the rabbit becomes a hare. So it seems with the battle between Hollywood, Florida and Hollywood, California. Low-carb guru Dr. Atkins, cardiologist from California, versus low-carb guru Dr. Agatston, cardiologist from Florida. Like Taco Bell and Taco Time, these two diets have a comparable slant on the same theory, with a few modifications. Unlike Dr. Atkins, Dr. Agatston has not died of heart disease and appears to be alive and well. Unlike the Atkins diet, SBD (South Beach Diet) promotes and encourages an increase of unsaturated and monounsaturated fats and a decrease in saturated fats. It also heavily restricts carbohydrates but more specifically high gly-cemic carbohydrates that tend to produce a severe insulin re-sponse in the body. Lastly, although the SBD restricts fruits and vegetables, it does encourage limited amounts of fibrous fruits and veggies such as apples, avocados and broccoli, based on their low glycemic rating.

Regurgitating the Atkins diet, the SBD is broken down into three fun-filled phases beginning with the, sum up your will-power because you're-going-to-need-it-like-you've-never-needed-it-before-unless-you-were-on-the-cabbage-soup-diet, phase. In this phase the Die with a t basically eliminates all brain food in the hopes of either breaking your spirit or your fluctuating blood sugar cycles. No fruit, no alcohol, no bread, no milk, no pasta, no rice, no sugar, no life, no sleep, no energy, no concentration. If you make it through phase one, which many of the reviews I read either gave up on or skipped, according to the book, you will be eight to 13 pounds lighter than you were two weeks ago. My gently sarcastic mind rolled these numbers around like dice, hoping to come up with a pair but inevitably ending up with a seven. No matter how you look at it, a loss of eight to 13 pounds is 28,000 to 45,500 calories, either eliminated or expended. Knowing how most people, caught on the diet treadmill, approach weight loss, I simply could not see the loss coming from the latter. South Beachers, weighing 160 pounds, would have to walk a 20-minute mile for 87-142 hours, in two weeks, in order to burn off those calories. So that, I said to my gently-sarcastic-self, must mean they had to decrease their calories between 2,000-3,250 calories per day to accomplish that kind of weight loss.

For most dieters, that would surely mean they were fasting. So, how then could they possibly lose that much weight in such a short period of time? Let's think for a second. Every gram of glucose (carbohydrates broken down into sugar) binds with three grams of water, so that must mean that every gram of glucose burned off or eliminated eliminates three grams of water. Tick tock, tick tock, tick tock..... kuku, kuku, kuku, that must mean they are losing huge amounts of water and perhaps some lean tissue too! That's great, as long as the scale is counting backwards, who cares?

Phase two and phase three were essentially the same as the Atkins plan. Reintroduce foods back into the diet, as long as the weight loss continues and until you reach your goal weight— whatever that was and wherever that came from— finally ending with a new variety of foods designed to maintain your goal weight for life.

What did I think of this program? Well, I'm not a cardiologist, I am just a chick who has been exposed to a thing or two about weight loss, but I can't help but wonder why a heart doctor would come up with a weight loss program that has little emphasis on exercise. One measly page in his book. I also wondered about the claims that you won't be hungry on this diet, and if you do get hungry, simply count out 15 cashews and enjoy them slowly. After I got up from falling off my chair with laughter, I looked up testimonials and noticed how many people complained about being hungry, nauseous and fatigued. I thought to myself, why not just count out 15 cashews and enjoy them slowly?

Next was the claim that the majority of the weight loss experienced on the SBD, was from the starving individual's midsection. If you carry 50 or 60 extra pounds around your midsection and have legs like a chicken riding a bike, it is obvious that you're going to see significant weight loss from your midsection. Dr. Agatston should shed some light on the mistaken belief that it is possible to spot reduce through dieting. Lastly, I found the lack of emphasis on portion control disturbing. It doesn't matter how healthy you eat, if you eat too much and you don't burn it off, it will get stored as fat. To say to a person that has been overeating for 20 years, "Just eat until full", is like telling an alcoholic to only drink until they feel a little bit drunk. Portion control is essential to weight loss and without guidance most people have no idea what a *normal size portion* looks like or what *eat until you're full*, means.

Should this diet be taken seriously? Absolutely. Contrary to what my tender mockery may imply, it has great merit in specific situations. Sadly, what Dr. Agatston designed this diet for is what it should be used for—people with diabetes, heart disease and other life-threatening health problems—not people who have already been beaten down by the diet industry. The concepts behind the *South Beach Diet* are scientific and clinically proven for certain demographics. It has great recipes and provides a vegetarian option. You don't have to buy pre-packaged foods that are supplied by the company and there is no journaling, counting or tracking. There are no prayer meetings or one-on-one counseling and there are no contracts binding you until death-do-us-part.

I believe if people are looking for a flexible, healthy nutrition plan, this may be an option, but they should seriously question phase one. They should commit to exercising on a daily basis and learn to recognize what full feels like and they should keep in mind that any low calorie diet will work if enough willpower is summoned. If you are going to attempt the SBD, my recommendation would be to record body fat percentages and not weight loss. If your body fat percentage is going up, but your weight is going down, you are losing muscle and water and not fat. Like any other weight loss program available, research the concepts, don't read the testimonials on the program's website. If it makes sound sense to you and you believe you can eat that way for life, then give it a try—at the very least, your heart will be happy.

The Zone Diet—Barry Sears, PhD, takes the emphasis off of carbohydrate reduction by putting the focus on increasing protein and fat intake. Shrewd. He suggests we think of food not as "a source of calories, but as a control system for hormones." That is like suggesting we think of sex as a way to make babies instead of a way to feel physical intimacy with our mate. Regardless, Mr. Sears is suggesting that we decrease our carbohydrate intake to 40 per cent of our dietary intake which is approximately 20 per cent less than the RDA but considerably more than the carbohydrate-cutting diets that have already been discussed. Obviously with a 20 per cent reduction in carbohydrate intake, we must have an increase in our protein and fat consumption. Luckily most people eat plenty of fat, so there is a good chance you are already at the 30 per cent fat intake. It is the protein that tends to be out of alignment with proper caloric consumption. This diet recommends a protein intake of 30 per cent of your daily caloric intake.

Although this type of mathematical eating can be a bit daunting, I like to make it simple by suggesting that every time you eat, consider what percentage of what you're eating is a carbohydrate, what percentage is a fat and what percentage is a protein. Tough if you don't know a protein from a carbohydrate but in general this does tend to simplify the process. If you are eating a steak, a baked potato with butter, sour-cream and chives, broccoli with cheese sauce and garlic bread, simply look at your plate and imagine what percentage comes from what. Steak is protein and fat, a baked potato is a carbohydrate, butter and sour-cream are fat and protein, chives and broccoli are carbohydrates, cheese sauce is fat and protein, and garlic bread is a carbohydrate and fat. This particular meal is heavy on the protein and fat and moderate on the carbohydrates.

I have to admit that I like the way this diet promotes the combination of proteins and carbohydrates in order to slow down the rate which insulin is produced. The premise behind this diet is to create a balanced physiological state within the body through hormone regulation. This delicate state is regulated by hormones such as insulin and eicosanoids, which are controlled by the foods we eat. The diet is designed to place the body within zones that are not too high and not too low, hence the name, *The Zone*. According to Sears, the benefits of controlling insulin levels are—increased fat loss, decreased likelihood of cardiovascular disease and greater physical and mental performance. The benefits to controlling eicosanoids are decreased inflammation and increased blood flow.

Although this diet draws mixed reviews from nutrition experts, some of the claims are easy to prove. Have you ever noticed when you eat an apple for a snack, it makes you burp, and then 20 minutes later you are hungry again? Try eating an apple with a couple of slices of low fat cheese or a handful of almonds and notice the apple will last much longer in your system. This is because the protein that you have combined with the apple helps to decrease the rate at which insulin is produced and absorbed, therefore, giving a longer feeling of satiety. I like the fact this diet promotes carbohydrate intake through fruits and vegetables and suggests reducing pasta, rice and breads, but not eliminating them. It discourages saturated fats and highly recommends supplementing with heart-healthy mono-unsaturates. Although it is a higher protein diet, it is not ridiculously high enough to produce a state of ketosis. Protein sizes are limited to approximately three ounces per meal for women and four ounces per meal for men. Dr. Sears also recommends keeping your caloric intake to 500 calories per meal and 100 calories per snack.

Although I was not offended by this particular program, there seemed to be a lot of professionals who were. They were, however, saying the same basic things about *The Zone* as they were about other low carbohydrate diets. Poor mental function, ketosis, lack of fruits and vegetables, too much fat, low calorie, etc. I didn't find this particular diet quite as ridiculous as the ultra-low carbohydrate diets. I did question the scientific way the book was written. It makes for a very difficult read for the average person who just wants some simple food guidelines without the thesis. Should you try it? Research the program and determine whether it fits your lifestyle, your natural food choices and if you can include it in your life, for life.

Protein Power—I have to say this is becoming a bit like playing the same record over and over and over until you want to place it gently under the back tire of your vehicle. Low-carb, high protein, various phases of elimination, ketosis, insulin, melt-away the pounds, this is the diet for you, Barry Sears praises it, nutrition experts pooh-pooh it. The only glaring difference that I could distinguish was the fact it was written by a husband *and* wife team of doctors, who recommend you drink a bit of alcohol each day, increase your fluid intake by as much as 50 per cent, and strongly suggest you include a vitamin/mineral supplement. For anyone with the slightest aptitude for critical thinking, these recommendations should throw up red flags. A bit of alcohol each day—everything in moderation except cocaine and heroin. Increase your fluid intake by as much as 50 per cent per day and start wearing Depends. A vitamin supplement should only be prescribed for people who are not able to consume the appropriate amount of nutrients through food variety. Even with a multi-vitamin, there are plenty of micronutrients in foods that we cannot get from supplements—we must get them through foods. This diet is based on the same principles as the rest of the high protein diets just with a different cover.

The GI Diet—This refers to the *Glycemic Index Diet*, which is once again another version of limiting your carbohydrate intake and replacing "bad carbs" with "good carbs". I was hoping for just one interesting diet, like, *Eat For Your Color Diet*. This diet would take scientific research, based on your favorite color, and produce statistics that show if you only eat foods from your favorite color palette, you are sure to melt away the pounds. Lucky you if you love the color green but not so lucky if your favorite color is blue. On Sundays you can add in one primary color and on the first Monday of each month you get to combine food colors as long as you never eat anything white. That would be fun!

The glycemic index is what low-carbohydrate, high protein diets are based on. This particular diet just gives you the actual glycemic index value of foods, which I believe is essential to making educated food choices.

When reading my obvious mockery towards these diets, keep in mind that I do believe there is a time, and a place for certain eating plans, for certain people. What I don't appreciate is every Dr. Tom, Dr. Dick and Dr. Harry writing a book, saying the same thing as 20 other books, and getting rich off your desperation. People would be better off taking their diet books to the secondhand store and replace them with books on nutrition, exercise, self-love, self-esteem, principles of effectiveness and critical thinking. Replace television with reading and with activity. This would empower both women and men to take back control from the diet industry. This would eliminate the *hope* factor and replace it with the *reality* factor. People would quit rubbing their thighs in the hopes that Aladdin would pop out of the next can of *Slim Fast*, and produce immediate, lasting results. Knowledge is power. The more people know and understand about how their body works and responds to imposed stresses, the better the chance they will treat it the way it was meant to be treated. With kindness. With respect. With forgiveness.

When I was researching information for this chapter I was astonished by the sheer number of diets that were available.

Two hundred and forty-seven on one particular website. I still wanted to be in my early 40s when this book was completed, so I wasn't able to research them all, but I felt compelled to list my favorites, based solely on name, along with my slow-witted commentary, for your sheer entertainment.

1 Day Diet—Great the day before a wedding or a reunion.
3 or 4 Day Diet—I prefer 3, thank you.
7 day diet—Getting a bit long for me.
5 Day Miracle—If you lose any weight, it will be a miracle.
8 Minutes in the Morning—Of what?
24 Hour Diet—Military version of the 1 day diet.
Abs Diet—You have them anyway, they are just hiding underneath some insulation.
Anorex—This is a great diet if you are already 50 pounds **underweight**.
Apple Cider Vinegar Diet—This diet turns you into a sour puss.
The Business Plan for the Body—Requires a shredder, a day planner and a palm pilot.
Cabbage Soup Diet—Keep in mind how gaseous cabbage can be.
Cactus Diet—Tough to chew and hard to swallow.
Carb Away—Sounds like something a wizard would say while waving his crooked wand.
Carb Blockers—Sounds like a patch worn to curb sugar cravings. Hey, that is a good idea!
Carb Cutters—Sounds like a mechanic's tool.
Carb Eliminator—Sounds like something the doctor would ask you to do in a small plastic cup.
Carbo Lock—Sounds like something off of Star Trek.
Celebrity Diets—Liposuction.
Chocolate Diet—By far the most popular diet.
Diet Power—This program comes with a superhero costume

designed to melt away calories.

Diet Teas—I hate tea.

The Eclipse—Close your eyes while doing this one. If you blink, you'll miss it.

The Egg Diet—Eggs for breakfast, eggs for lunch and a sensible meal for dinner.

Fat Flush Plan—Takes place in the bathroom.

French Women's Diet—Calories are counted in French to make it sound more romantic.

Grapefruit Diet—For variety combine with the egg, cabbage soup, cactus and chocolate diets.

Hawaii Diet—Doesn't work well if you live somewhere cold.

Hollywood Diets—Liposuction, plastic surgery, diet pills and anti-depressants.

Hollywood 48 Hour Miracle Diet—This happens at the Betty Ford Clinic.

Ice Cream Diet—Combine with egg, cabbage soup, cactus, grapefruit and chocolate diets.

Idiot Proof Diet—Who are you calling an idiot?

Lap Band—Makes me think of a stripper dancing on my lap.

The Laze Diet System—Great for people who don't like to exercise, shop or eat healthy.

Miami Diet—The South Beach Diet versus Dr. Atkins. Hawaii versus Miami.

 Mommy Style—Move home, regardless of your age.

Negative Calorie Diet—You only eat foods you dislike.

One Day Diet—This is the long version of the 1 Day Diet.

Peel Away the Pounds—While sitting in our patented fat jiggler suit—yours for only $2000.

Personality Type Diet—Don't even get me started on this one.

Popcorn Diet—You have to watch a lot of DVDs to enjoy this diet.

Reverse Diet—Overeating and no exercise is the key to this diet.

Rice Diet—You won't hear Dr. Atkins or Dr. Agatston supporting this diet.

Skinny Pill—It is really small.

Skinny Pill for Kids—This one is even smaller.

Sleep A-Weigh—When you wake up you haven't gained a pound since last night.

Subway Diet—Not to be confused with the McDonald's Diet or the Wendy's Diet.

T-Burn Fat Attack Combo—T-bone steaks, French fries and a large coke constitute this diet.

Tony Little's Gazelle—This was supposed to be listed under—*Famous People and their Pets.*

Ultimate Carb Phaser 1000—Weighs 680 pounds and takes three days to put together.

Utah Diet—Not great if you live in Idaho.

You on a Diet—Poor English for, "Would you like to go on a diet?"

I hope this chapter encourages you to stop participating in what others tell you will work and persuades you to start learning what will work best for you.

Simple weight loss information.

When you are reading through these reviews don't get mad at me for criticizing your favorite diet. I invite you to take the information from this chapter and apply it to your favorite diet and see if it fits the criteria for a healthy approach to weight loss. Does it recommend activity and exercise on a regular basis? Does it eliminate food groups? Does it outline portion sizes and snacks? Does it include nutrient-dense foods such as vegetables, fruits and whole grains? Does it satisfy you? Is it manageable? Is it realistic? Can you include this way of eating in your life, for life?

Be responsible for your weight-loss choices. Read as much as you can about a diet, preferably not on their website as they tend to be biased. Talk to a dietician or a nutritionist. Talk to people who have tried the program. Look up long term results on the Internet. Don't take the information that is being shoved at you as gospel. Anyone can write a diet book or develop a diet plan or invent a diet pill but that doesn't mean they will work. What works for one person does not necessarily mean it will work for you. Be smart and get educated about the program you choose.

6
MEDIA

The media is a corporate world that makes money off un-conscious thinking. It trains us to think with our wallet instead of our minds. Young girls today are hit the hardest. They are taught and trained to believe they will be popular and sexy and successful if they just buy the right jeans, wear the right mascara and listen to the right music. They also need to eat at the right fast food restaurant and order the latest "right choice". They are taught that sex sells alcohol. That cars spell success. That money equals happiness. That happiness can be bought with just the right perfume, skin cream and lipstick. They are suffering and struggling with the splitting of their personalities into their old-self and their new-self. Their old-self knows that mascara doesn't make you happy but their new-self thinks it will make them pretty and *pretty* makes you happy. They haven't traveled far enough down the road of wisdom to realize that happiness can only be found one short turn to the left of the soul.

Some of us never travel far enough down that road to find the street sign that reads "happiness" so we keep taking the turns we think are going to bring us home. Those turns are named after perfume companies and jean companies and car companies and diet companies.

Magazines teach us that women are objects that can be bought. They teach us that half-naked bodies of women sell male products. Makes sense that a beautiful blonde woman in a beer label bathing suit would sell a tractor—men think the blonde comes with the tractor. Half-naked women grinding their pelvis to rock n' roll while men watch and drool, will sell more beer because we are taught to believe if we buy the right brand of beer, the opposite sex will pop out of the can. I recently flipped through one of our son's car magazines to get a feel for how far companies will go to sell their products. By the end of the magazine, I realized I was looking at a soft porn magazine. Fifty-two ads using all-but-naked women to sell their products. Words like ecstasy, headers, Xplod, SEMA, Shining Monkey, pure, and HOT, sealing the fate of every libido-driven man to buy because we all know that, not only does the naked girl come with the product, she'll install it for you too! Women's bodies are used and abused in every way to sell products—bondage, pornography, vulnerable positions, sex trafficking, heroin-addict thin, naked, abuse. The media will depict women in any manner to sell product.

The media dictates what it takes to be *beautiful*, to be *successful*, to be *happy*. Heroin addict thin is beautiful. The $60,000 car, in *BLACK*, means you have found success. Being heroin-addict thin with an expensive car means a future full of happiness. Wouldn't it be interesting to know how many women working in the media selling us this mind-litter have bought into their own fantasy?

We know that once our daughters hit adolescence, many times we as the parents are no longer their primary influence. Instead young girls start watching and emulating their friends, and their friends get their ideas and messages from the mass media. According to statistics on the Internet, the average teen watches approximately 21 hours of television each week, compared to 5.8 hours spent on homework and 1.8 hours spent reading. Our daughters are being brought up and influenced by an electronic society that includes rap music, television, videos, cell phones, MSN, I-Pods, the Internet and movies. Allowing our children to live in this society is scary and risky at best. Cool, as presented by the media, implies drinking, violence, inappropriate language, spending money and being sexually active. We think because our kids participate in this society in the safety of our own homes, they are safe. Big mistake. Look at what your kids' friends are writing about on MSN. Listen to the words of the music they listen to. Watch the music videos they love. Sit and watch the weekly shows they enjoy on general cable. Watch the movies they are getting their ideas from. Check the history on your Internet and see where they have been surfing. You will be hard-pressed to find a music video of their genre that is not soft porn. It teaches our daughters that this is an acceptable way to dress and conduct themselves if they want to be popular and have a boyfriend. Check out the way they talk to each other on MSN. They may not be verbalizing the foul language they are hearing on television, in movies, and in music, but they sure have no problem typing it. They will tell the boys on MSN that they love them like it's a new flavor of ice-cream. They say stuff over the computer that they would never say to each other face to face because the impersonal nature of the computer gives them courage. They are becoming de-sensitized to language, sex, violence, and pornography. They are losing respect for themselves and for others. They don't understand the concept of working hard for money and their general attitude is one of—everyone has one so I deserve one too. Gone are the days of the *Fresh Prince of Bel-Air, Full House, Indiana Jones, The Flintstones, Looney Tunes*. Here to stay are *The Simpsons*, reality television (heaven help us), *The Simple Life, South Park, Trailer Park Boys, Much Music*, and *Sex in the City*.

Someone once said to me that it was ridiculous to not let our son have cable television, MSN, a cell phone, a computer in his room or a Game Boy. She felt that children today are being raised in an electronic society and their entire futures will be conducted in an electronic society, so why fight it. I say, when the day comes that there is no longer a phone, he can have MSN. When he can afford to buy his own cable, his own computer and pay his own cell phone bill, then go for it. Until then, one family computer, one family television and a damn telephone. He has lived for 14 years without cable television, without MSN, and without a Game Boy.

For his 13th birthday we bought him a television for his room and for Christmas of his 13th year, we bought him a Play Station. We bought into the media hype. Big mistake. Now where does he spend his time? In his room. What does he like to do? Play video games. If we got MSN, where would he be? On the computer. For 14 years we watched four channels on a 27-inch Sears television with rabbit ears. He drew, he played, he hung out with his friends, he acted like a kid. Now when his buddies come over, they head upstairs and sit down in front of the Play Station, allowing their brains leak into cyberspace. It is said that the technological advancements that are available to our kids today are making them dumber. They don't know how to sit and read a book. They don't know how to answer a telephone. They can't focus unless they are bombarded with noise and action. They can't have an intelligent conversation with an adult. They have difficulty communicating unless it involves cell phones, text messaging and MSN. This is the society our children are living in and being raised in. The media teaches them this is the norm and we provide them with the means.

Watch how many commercials are on television for Play Station, Game Cube, X-Box, I-Pod, Nano, Shuffle, the Chocolate, RAZR and SLVR cell phone, plasma televisions, flat screen televisions, MacIntosh computers, and computer capabilities. Now think about your daughters. Think about how we let them buy into all of the electronic buzz created by the media and ask yourself, 'If I let them buy into something that I can control, imagine how easy it is for them to buy into media concepts that I can't control'. Am I saying we shouldn't let our daughters watch television, go to movies or talk to their friends. Mmm, no. I am saying if you are going to encourage them to participate in this electronic age, don't blame the media for what they are learning. Take responsibility for where your daughters are finding their role models, learning many of their life lessons and establishing their priorities. It is not a blaming game, it is an accountability game.

The media has the goal of making money from humans, and teenagers are one of their prime targets. On the other hand, our primary goal as parents is to produce happy, well-adjusted, community-serving adults. These two goals are not compatible. Mothers tend to be confused, scared and frustrated by their daughters' media-induced values and this causes resistance and friction between them.

"If you dress and look like a movie star, everyone will like you and that will mean you are successful."

Interview client #16

"The media determines what is beautiful."
Interview client #47

"The media pushes—you are what you wear. When I don't feel good about my body and I am flipping through magazines looking at all the skinny women, it makes me feel even worse."
Interview client #46

"I know Photoshop and I know what can be done."
Interview client #22

Throughout many of my interviews it was interesting to observe one of the common threads that connected women together and it was their intolerance of being judged or compared. They felt wherever they went, people looked at them and snickered or stared or silently judged. As much as they hated it, they did it themselves. One woman openly admitted even though she was overweight and divorced and had not dated in 14 years, she would really have to suck it up to date a man that was overweight. She wanted what she saw on television and she believes men want what they see on television. The men on television are usually fit, healthy, groomed, and successful, unless it's a beer commercial. Women are usually thin, happy, beautiful, and coiffed. Have you ever seen the Swifter commercial where the woman is sweeping her kitchen in high heels, dress clothes and a great big smile? I don't know about you but I don't usually have a smile on my face when I have to sweep the floor regardless of how pretty the broom is.

"You can't win. Every time you turn on the television there is a food ad followed by a diet ad."   **Interview client #50**

"The media perpetuates everything but no matter how hard I try not to buy into the crap, I watch *America's Next Top Model* and I want to be just like them. I want to be skinny, beautiful, tall, blonde, and wear the clothes and be looked at. No matter how realistic I am, I can't help but wish it were true. It's terrible but beautiful." **Interview client #15**

"Fat equals ugly and thin equals beautiful. The media infers that only slim, beautiful people can be successful."
Interview client #51

"The media makes me think that skinny is beautiful and that altering it through plastic surgery is okay because 'everyone' is doing it." **Interview client #73**

"Media. It has created the evolution of women. At the same time it has helped us to evolve, it causes us the greatest regression. We have come so far in terms of our roles in life but with that comes a need to look better in order to feel worthy. It's what gets us through the door. Society is very vanity-oriented and much of that has to do with the media."
Interview client #20

"Between television, magazines and the Internet, one cannot keep up with the expectations of trying to age gracefully. In other words, the media exposes your small discomforts that you have surrounding your body image."
Interview client #68

"Anyone struggling with body image issues should start by avoiding all the advertising and propaganda!"
Interview client #55

"The media describes and prescribes ideal. It is all fantasy."
Interview client #64

"The media tries to make me and others feel that we are worthless because we are not thin."
Interview client #71

"I think it is so sad that the media tries to make us feel inadequate unless we are perfect in face and body."
Interview client #70

"It makes me want to spit. I'm furious. The media is killing people. It's unconscionable. It's irresponsible and it's responsible for death."
Interview client #39

"The media pushes, 'you are what you look like'."
Interview client #46

We are constantly bombarded with advertisements that make everything look beautiful and easy, simple and clean. We see advertisements for quick, easy and enjoyable solutions to the weight loss dilemma but we rarely see ads promoting easy, quick and enjoyable solutions to alcoholism, gambling or drugs. We know that once we kick those habits we never have to go back to them, but it's not so easy with food addictions because we can't live without food. Advertisements for food addictions should be as serious and depressing as the ones for AA, Alanon, and Gamblers Anonymous because it is the worst substance to be addicted to. We can never live without it therefore we have to learn to make peace with it.

Food exploits our weakness.

According to the video, *A Matter of Fat*, more than $425 million are spent advertising food each year in Canada, $36 billion in the U.S. The four most advertised foods are fast food, high-sugar cereal, pop and candy. The video also states there are currently eight million obese people in Canada and that number is doubling every seven years.

According to a study by Harrison and her colleagues out of the University of Illinois at Urbana-Champaign, many television ads for unhealthy foods are targeted at our kids. The study found that 44 per cent of ads aired during children's programs aged 6-11, were for high-sugar foods, and that 34.2 per cent of television ads were for fast foods. The study also found that snack time eating was more prominently displayed than traditional meal times. The eating locations depicted in ads were outdoors or in cars. Harrison and her colleagues determined that, on average, about 10.65 food ads air per hour in their study's sample size. Previous research had found that pre-teens watch about three hours of television a day. This translates into 11,000 food ads watched by each pre-teen a year.

We are inundated, on a daily basis, with ads on television and in print, about food. Snickers is a healthy snack because it has peanuts. A&W is a classy, romantic place to go for a burger. McDonald's serves healthy food that makes you happy. Fruit roll-ups are a healthy snack because they start with the word fruit. Frosted Flakes taste great therefore they must be great. Nutella is a healthy choice, rich in protein and vitamins. If I saw those ads 11,000 times a year, I might begin to believe them too. It comes down to education. Just because someone tells you that taking this little blue pill will eliminate your chances of cancer, doesn't mean you are going to take it. You would research the product and the company first. You would contact the Better Business Bureau and perhaps the FDA. Talk to past and present clients, research the side effects, determine how long the company has been in business and so on and so on. It should be the same with food products. Just because a food product says it is organic doesn't mean that it is a better option. Just because whole milk has Vitamin A and D doesn't mean it is the right choice for you. Just because a fruit drink says it has Vitamin C, doesn't mean you should be drinking it. Just because potato chips say they are now unsaturated, doesn't mean they are healthy.

I have noticed a subtle change in the way the media is defining beautiful and I can't help but wonder if the pressure the media has created to be thin, is starting to backfire and it is being forced to back pedal, like a swimmer away from a water snake. In the past six months ultra-thin models Luisel Ramos, 22, and Ana Carolina Reston, 21, died of complications surrounding their anorexia. In September of 2006, Madrid banned five models from the catwalks for being too thin. It was determined that a BMI of less than 18 would not be permitted in the show. This is due to a growing alarm surrounding the ultra-thin, ultra-unhealthy look that is being promoted by the fashion industry and the media and is being emulated by young girls around the world.

Dove is taking the world by storm with their *Campaign for Real Beauty* which promotes and encourages beauty from within not from without. Tyra Banks is standing up to the media and is saying, "I'm not fat." Plus size models are becoming just as famous as their size zero (who wants to be known as a zero anyway?) counterparts. Queen Latifah, Beyonce, Mariah Carey, Jennifer Hudson, America Ferrera, Tyra Banks and Oprah Winfrey are encouraging women to embrace their curves. Segments of the fashion industry are starting to revolt against the ultra-thin models. Movie stars such as the Olsen twins, Nicole Richie, Victoria Beckham and Keira Knightley, are being openly scorned for their drastic weight loss and heroine-addict appearance.

Has society finally had enough of the dung the media is spoon feeding them? I don't think our appetite for Hollywood gossip will ever be satiated but I do believe women are starting to wake up from their sugar-induced comas and are beginning to realize that it is all just a fantasy. Those beautiful big lips, those perfect upright breasts, that flawless complexion, the cottage cheese-free thighs, the grey-free hair, the perfect chicklet teeth, the flab-free abs, the ass like a ballerina, the 42 carat princess cut diamond, the $1,500 socks, the $400 bum thong in every color, the white Mercedes for Monday and the tan Benz for Tuesday, the perfect husband with the perfect teeth and the washboard abs, the darling little dog that looks like a rat with a mane, wearing more jewels than we will ever own, the 238 pairs of shoes, Christmas in Cabo San Lucas, New Years in Maui, Valentine's Day in the South Pacific, and so on and so on and so on. It is unrealistic and ridiculous.

What do we enjoy most about all of this Hollywood entertainment? When it falls apart and movie stars are left exposed and vulnerable like the rest of us. It allows the general public to realize it doesn't matter how rich you are, how beautiful you are or how successful you are, you are not immune to the sadness, illness, weakness, frustration, heartbreak and death that the rest of the world is exposed to. The bigger the fame, the further the fall.

I believe there is tremendous opportunity for positive initiative through the media but it is up to us to utilize and maximize the media for personal growth not personal misery. We should take full advantage of our ability to access information through various medium in order to move us toward our goal of a better life and a better world, not let it suck us into a void of unconsciousness, misery and greed.

7
MOTHERS

"And the sins of the fathers are visited on the children for generations and generation." Unknowingly taking on our parent's unresolved issues can lead to the passing on of dysfunctional habits. Time and time again we are set up to take on our parent's unresolved issues without even knowing it. My father was an alcoholic and his father was an alcoholic and his father was an alcoholic. My mother was fat and her mother was fat and her mother was fat. My father beat my mother and my mother's father beat his wife and my husband beats me.

Many of the women that I interviewed learned their dysfunctional habits from their mothers. They learned to self-loath, to people-please, to be pretty and quiet, to place men before themselves, to place children before themselves, to question their self-worth, to avoid feelings such as anger, fear or sadness and they learned how to diet. Up until about the age of five, most of what children do and think comes from the primitive area of their brain that just knows how to survive.

Blink, breathe, cry, smile, fart, digest, move away from painful stimulus, sleep, pee, eat. Everything else is learned from our external existence. We start with empty mega-bites.

For example, when a child cries, generally speaking, we do everything we can to stop the child from crying and very often it is done with food. Slowly, over time, a child learns that being unhappy or being uncomfortable can be soothed with food. Taught not inherent. Putting fingernail polish on your child at the age of three teaches them that being pretty is important. Telling your daughter that she is looking chubby teaches her she is fat. Constantly criticizing the way you look teaches your daughter to self-loath. Constantly making comments about having to lose weight teaches our daughters to diet. And so the brain starts to fill up with all sorts of messages influenced by friends and family and the media. The bits of information storing on our mental hard-drive—one negative message at a time—until eventually we become just like the messages we have stored away. Sad, angry, anxious, unhappy, afraid, uncertain and jealous.

Puberty

The relationship between mothers and daughters can be like a war zone, especially during puberty. The child wants so badly to continue to be a child and to be mommy's little girl but everything in society teaches her that she needs to break away from mommy's apron strings and become a "woman". She needs to dress a certain way, she needs to think a certain way, she needs to look a certain way and she needs to act a certain way. Gone are the days of being completely content with who she is/was and here to stay are the days of *doing* and *being* exactly what society deems acceptable. The start of questioning: Am I good enough? Do I look good enough? Will he/she like me? Am I going to fail? Am I fat? Am I pretty?

As the mother of one 14-year-old son and no daughters, this project has been enlightening. I was a young girl once and obviously went through puberty, but seemed to breeze through it with little to no trauma. I also had two younger sisters that I thought breezed through puberty although I can't be certain. I realize now that puberty sets the framework for the young women that girls become.

Their ability to make informed decisions starts with us. Their level of self-confidence starts with us. Their learned nutritional habits start with us. Their ability to communicate starts with us. Their ability to self-nurture and self-love starts with us. Their ability to diet starts with us. If we only knew, going into motherhood, just how difficult the job of MOTHER truly would be. How incredibly important it is for us to be mentally healthy before submitting our children to our lack of mental health. What it is like to be needed 24/7. Some women think that is the answer to their acquired emptiness. The more they focus their attention on helping everyone around them the less they have to help themselves. They spend their whole day in a tornado of tasks meant to improve everyone else's life in order to avoid the storm raging inside themselves. The irony is in the improving of everyone else's life. We learned this from our upbringing and we are teaching it to our daughters and they will teach it to their daughters just like an alcoholic teaches their child and a man who beats his wife teaches his child.

"My father was an alcoholic and beat my mother. Neither of them was ever there for me emotionally. I quite often ended up taking care of my siblings and wished for the day that I would meet a man that would marry me so we could have kids.

I would never, ever treat them the way my parents treated me!" Sound familiar? This is the type of little girl that places all her emphasis on finding a man. In order to do that, she has to look a certain way and act a certain way. This attracts a certain type of mate, which really doesn't matter because she will take whatever she can get in order to get away from where she is. Now it's too late. She is pregnant, living in a run-down mobile home, working the night shift at a gas station while her boyfriend goes out drinking and partying with his buddies until the early morning hours. The cycle begins again and again, and again.

Interview client #47's mother once told her that if she didn't like her weight the way it was, she could just stick a pencil down her throat.

We created ourselves in a manner that we thought would bring us all the riches in the world. A husband, children, a successful career, a nice house, a white picket fence, a nice car. In the process of attempting to achieve the "All American Dream", we lost our self along the way. A life of uncertainty is the price we pay for second rate love. Often, this trade-off for love occurs firstly with our relationships with our mothers. We take what we learn from them into our adult life. We want so badly to be loved but we desperately need our independence. We struggle with so many fears and we deal with them by eating. Eating keeps us from feeling what we have created. If we take our focus off of our obsession with food and with being thin, we have to deal with how much of ourselves we have lost in order to play the "All American Dream".

Listening to the young girls in elementary school, it was obvious that the "All American Dream" had not yet occurred. They didn't care about love or about boys or about a future career. They were living in the moment and they loved being in the moment. The majority of the young girls picked their moms as their role models. Their role models were loving, helpful, caring and always made things better. On the other hand, somewhere between the spring of Grade 6 and the fall of Grade 7, the girls had their priorities flipped around like a drunken gymnast. In elementary school they could talk to their moms about anything but in middle school—more so Grades 8 and 9—the girls didn't feel that they could tell their moms everything. When I asked who they would talk to if they had a problem, they typically answered their friends. I thought, Dear God, hormone number one is counseling hormone number two on the fine art of kissing and how to deal with her period!

Because I said so, that's why!

If we want our girls to start loving their bodies, we have to start by loving ours. We need to start taking the focus away from how we look on the outside and redirect it at how we feel on the inside. We need to minimize the emphasis that we place on our appearance and start to redirect it at how we are feeling. If we, as mothers, want to raise healthy, happy daughters, we have to start with ourselves. If we don't eat breakfast, we can't preach to our daughters to eat breakfast. If we constantly self-loath, we can't tell them how they look doesn't matter because they are perfect the way they are. If we are constantly on a diet, we shouldn't be surprised when they try their first diet at age 11.

One of the women I interviewed had suffered for years with severe dysfunctional eating habits. She was very open and painfully honest about her unhappiness with her marriage, her feelings of inadequacy with her family, her lack of self-worth and her dysfunctional food habits. When I asked her how she felt it was affecting her two teen daughters, she replied, "They don't have any idea what I am going through. I make a point of sheltering them from my habits and talk to them constantly about their body and their health. I always make sure I have an excuse for my behavior and my actions." Wouldn't it be interesting to interview the two daughters?

"When I was in my late teens, early 20s, my mom kept trying to put me on a diet because she was slim and she thought I wasn't." **Interview client #62**

"My mother was very overweight and I watched her struggle with it since I was a little girl. She tried everything to lose weight but she dealt with life by eating." **Interview client #50**

"My mother was always critical of my appearance and my weight." **Interview client #60**

"My mother always told me it was inside that counts." **Interview client #30**

"I don't want my struggle with food and weight to become my daughter's struggle." **Interview client #20**

"My mother is four foot ten and 40 pounds overweight. As a kid, she was always on some sort of diet and encouraged me to participate. Diet Centre, TOPS, grapefruit diet, etc. She used to suffer from anorexia and at the age of 62, she still suffers with body image and weight issues." **Interview client #47**

"My mother started it all!" **Interview client #46**

"Hmmm—my mother has made the biggest (negative) impact in my life. It is such a huge issue that it could be the subject of a book in itself." **Interview client #13**

"My mom was always going on Weight Watchers whenever she wanted to look great for a wedding or a holiday or an event." **Interview client #41**

"All of the girls in my family have healthy self-esteem but my mom doesn't and she tries to deflect her low self-esteem back on us girls. She was always a great baker and used to use her baking as a reward or as a celebration." **Interview client #24**

"When we were kids, my mother was a real cooker. She used food as a coping mechanism. Now she is an enabler. When I am trying to lose weight, she will say, 'dessert?'. My mom is still very overweight and she judges other people that are overweight. She likes it when my sister and I gain weight." **Interview client #16**

"When I was growing up, we ate large amounts of unhealthy food. When we were unhappy, we ate." **Interview client #42**

"So far my daughter appears to be okay. I am very aware of what I say and do around her so she doesn't end up with my issues." **Interview client #12**

"Mom started restricting my calories when I was 18 months old so that I didn't get fat. She herself was very overweight. To this day she won't talk about it because she is in denial." **Interview client #38**

"My mother had a huge impact on my weight and my food issues. We were constantly getting mixed messages. She would say that I was fat and needed to lose weight but she would always be baking and allowed me to eat it."

Interview client #11

Nurture and nourish.

Moms are the best. Their internal desire to protect and nurture comes from thousands of years of primal nurturing passed down from generation to generation. They have an inherit longing to place their children's priorities and needs before theirs. Without moms, the world would be a loveless place and children would wither from emotional malnourishment. I am not implying all moms should get the *Betty Crocker Golden Seal of Approval* or dads can't be equally as nurturing but in general, children have a bond with their mothers that is unlike any other bond between two humans.

Unfortunately moms can't be everything and they can't do everything. They wear too many hats and place too high an expectation on themselves. Their lives tend to be fueled by guilt, pressure, stress and fatigue and this often spills over onto the people closest to them. They try so hard to accomplish the "super mom" status that they lose themselves and become someone entirely different from who they once were. You often hear comments such as, "I used to be so much fun", "I didn't use to be like this", "I don't know what happened to me", "Where did I go", "I wish I could be like the old me", "I remember when I used to like doing that", "She is not the woman I married". How could she be? When she got married, she was confident, independent, career-oriented, fun-loving, a social butterfly, thin, pretty, rested, unscheduled, carefree, adventurous, exciting, and happy.

Today moms work, raise children, volunteer, maintain a home, and attempt to be present and accountable in a marriage. But society doesn't think this is enough anymore. Now it's not just that they work but what they do that is important. Not only are they trying to raise children, but raising your child has become a competition. Ballet Monday through Friday, voice lessons on Tuesday and Thursday, tutoring on Saturday, rep soccer Monday, Wednesday, Saturday and Sunday, piano on Friday and Monday and swim lessons on Tuesday. If moms think they're tired, imagine how tired their children are. Like so many facets of life, being a mom and a wife has become a subliminal game of comparing and judging that leaves women with a sense of never quite measuring up. It's time to take the lid off the pressure cooker before it explodes leaving behind bits and pieces of a broken marriage, a shattered self-image and an empty life.

Moms need to realize just how important self-nourishment is for self-preservation. It is essential to their well-being and the well-being of those around them. Without self-nurturing, moms become an angry shell of sadness, fear, resentment, and frustration. These feelings chip away at their self-esteem and their self-worth making it impossible to love themselves. It is essential for moms to start taking the time they need to re-fuel and re-energize their bodies and their minds. An energized, relaxed woman is one who sees herself through happy, contented eyes and, in turn, is able to create a sense of well-being in her relationships and her surroundings. Being a mom is the toughest job a woman will ever have. It doesn't come with an owners' manual, directions, or a how-to DVD. It just comes with the primal knowledge of how to protect and nurture. Moms need to learn how to take care of themselves, guilt-free, so they have the mental and physical well-being to nurture and protect the ones they love.

Moms

We come into this world
and are touched by a soul,
whose love has no boundaries.

We are cuddled and coddled
suckled and soothed,
with the sway of pure contentment.

We grow and develop
learn and test,
knowing the arms of love
are forever nearby.

A lost tooth, a broken toy
a lost love, a broken heart,
never too tough
for her to soothe.

A smile,
a hug,
will wipe away tears
and make you wonder,
what was so wrong.

Time marches on,
a wrinkle appears,
her hands look different,
the odd grey hair.

You begin to wonder
what will it be like,
birthdays and Christmas,
when there is no mother.

No matter how hard you try
you just can't imagine,
for she has always been there,
and in your heart,
will be,
forever and ever.

Mia

8
DAUGHTERS

As I listened to the young girls for this book, I was enlight-ened by what a girl-corrupted culture we live in. The more I listened to them talk about their music, television, magazines, role models and movies and the more I looked at the sexist ad-vertising, the more I realized how set-up for low self-esteem our young girls are. The media today defines girls' develop-ment, limits their personalities and leaves many of them set up for depression, abuse and addiction.

I spent two days talking with and listening to 35 girls in Grades 4 through 6. I asked them 14 questions related to self-image, eating habits, goals, and role models. They also com-pleted a picture exercise, where they looked at various pictures of women and wrote down what came to mind. On the second day, we discussed the 14 questions and finished with a word association exercise. I held up various words and they wrote down what came to mind. Words such as bathing suit, food, the perfect you, your body.

The first thing I found so interesting was how hard they studied the pictures of the women. What they saw didn't seem to be immediate, they really had to look at the pictures in order to come up with something to write. The second thing was how many of them didn't even see the women. One picture was of a voluptuous woman holding a bowl of cherries and the majority of the girls commented on the cherries. Another picture was of Selma Hayek standing among some leaves and the girls commented more on the surroundings than on her. The last woman was a heavier-set woman in a business suit standing in a long hallway and many of the girls thought she was smart and rich but not necessarily heavy.

The girls were so eager to talk and to answer questions and were so open and honest that I was a little taken aback. They happily brought up subjects such as their periods, divorce, bras, middle school, and friends. At this age they didn't seem to notice or care if other girls were heavy or skinny, one young girl even commented that she thought the fatter girls were nicer and the skinny girls were snobby and she was a tall, thin, pretty young thing. Their biggest worry at this age was getting good grades and that their families were happy and healthy. They didn't care much about clothing, boys, food, diets, weight, makeup, hair or impressing anyone. They did like to look at their mother's and sister's magazines for the fashion *Dos and Don'ts* as well as the best and worst-dressed. Some of the Grade 5 and most of the Grade 6 girls admitted they already weighed themselves but didn't really know why. There were only two or three that weighed themselves because they wanted to know if they were gaining weight. They were polite, respectful and encouraging toward each other. They had simple goals, such as good grades or excelling at a sport. Twenty-three of the girls picked their mother as their role model, eight picked other members of their family and only four picked someone famous.

Most of the girls, even in Grade 4, knew what they wanted to be when they grew up. They picked careers such as professional athletes, teachers, pharmacists, veterinarians, marine biologists, singers, dancers, farmers, photographers, physiotherapists, artists, pediatric doctors. Some would indicate three or four different career paths. Wouldn't it be interesting to talk to these girls in three years and then five years and then 10 years to see if they are as confident as they are now?

The girls openly admitted that their moms talked about being fat and going on diets but they also admitted that almost as many fathers did as well. None of them thought their parents needed to diet and thought they were perfect the way they were. When we asked the group if they thought it was important to look a certain way or dress a certain way the girls didn't really see it as an issue. When the counselor, Lorri McPhee, asked one group, "Is it important to look like a model?" One young girl in Grade 6 stated, "It's ridiculous to feel like you have to look like the models in magazines." When McPhee asked what was important, she shrugged like we had both lost our marbles and said, "Saving the world, of course."

They loved to laugh and to chit-chat. They loved their families, their friends and their pets. School was very important to them and at this point was not a stressful place to be. They didn't appear to have issues with food or with their weight. The majority of the girls, even in Grade 6, had little interest in boys and looked at them more as friends.

Cut to the tween years.

I remember when I was a young girl in Grades 7 through

9 thinking everyone must be on drugs. It seemed the only logical answer to the way girls behaved. Girls were mean, spastic, loud, unstable, intense, volatile, secretive, anxious, uncommunicative, bi-polar, and arrogant. They lived in an altered state of reality that made them the centre of the universe and the one thing worth thinking about. When I looked up actions, symptoms and characteristics of someone on an LSD trip, it pretty much described adolescent girls. Keep in mind that they can also be kind, loving, nurturing and helpful—if it aligns with their universe.

The tween girls were the next group of girls I interviewed. Grades 7 through 9. It was obvious from the start that these girls were going to be much more reserved and were not going to volunteer any information that might not be considered the status quo. Their answers were influenced by what their friends thought, what their friends said, and how their friends acted. They didn't seem to have the confidence or the enthusiasm that the younger girls had.

When I asked them what they worried about, it was apparent that their concerns ran deeper than those of their younger fledglings. They worried about their parents divorcing, about cancer, about death in the family and about whether they would find a husband. They all worried about they way they looked and what people thought of them and they worried about being popular. Gone were the days of lying on their backs, on a warm summer day, turning the clouds into animals and fairies, with grass stains and milk moustaches. Here to stay were the formative days of confusion, frustration, anxiety, judging and comparing.

The tween girls had begun experimenting with make-up, with wearing a bra, with having a boyfriend, (no one seemed to be able to clarify exactly what the term boyfriend meant and I wasn't sure I wanted to know) and with dressing more seductively. They were in various stages of getting their first period and were very happy to share that information. When I was a young girl, bras, periods, and boys were secreted like a first kiss. Today they are paraded in front of us like a lottery winning in a gas station. When I was in school, the only time you saw a boy's underwear is when someone got a wedgie. Today, bras and underwear are meant to be exposed like a tattoo. Girls and boys hang all over their "date" like cats preening and having your period is like getting a raise—you make sure everyone knows about it.

The pressure for these girls to *be* is all-consuming. They have to be sexy. They have to be popular. They have to be skinny. They have to be funny. They have to be smart. They have to be pretty. They have to be good at sports. They have to be with a boy. They have to be dressed a certain way. Where did they learn the need to *be*? Society, media, family and friends. How do we prevent the pressure to *be*? I believe we start by trying not to *be* ourselves.

The big teens.

I was so impressed with this group of students. I'm not sure if I got an exceptional bunch of young people or if teenagers are just becoming more mature. Either way, what they shared was educational, informative, honest and wise. Let me start by saying this was a bit of a different experience for me because it was a group of 30 students, both male and female. Up to this point I had not included the male perspective in this journey—I figured the subject was complicated enough without adding another hormone into the mix. Regardless, the boys were in the group so I figured, what the heck, let's hear their perspective. It was a perspective worth mentioning.

I got the students to complete the same questions and the same exercises as the kids from Grades 4 through Grade 10. They took the questions seriously and provided me with very descriptive answers. As always, I began by asking them what they worried about to see how it compared with the younger kids. This age group worried mainly about their future career choices, about the stress of school work, tests and assignments and getting a part-time job.

They also worried about acceptance, family situations, friends, the opposite sex, appearance, death, and failing. They were no longer living in the moment, they were starting to live in the future and in the past.

The second concept I was most interested in comparing against the younger kids was the idea of a role model. Seven students didn't have one, three picked their mom, two picked their dad and two picked their sister. The rest looked at someone famous such as Pierre Trudeau, Tyra Banks or Hugh Laurie. I also wanted to know who and what motivated them.

"My expectations and the expectations of family, friends and teachers. When someone thinks highly of you, you want to remain in their good light and if they think poorly of you, you want to prove them otherwise."   **Student**

"My boyfriend. He knows exactly what he wants and who he is as a person. He does not fall under media or peer pressure. He has goals and a future. He is not self-conscious. He is my rock."   **Student**

"Independence."   **Student**

"My guilt, my parents, my friends and God. Generally, people I trust, because I know they care about me and want what's best for me." **Student**

"My family because they are there no matter how much I doubt myself." **Student**

"Parents and teachers because they make me realize that school is the stepping stone to my future life." **Student**

"My parents because impressing them is the most important thing for me to do." **Student**

"Extrinsic pressures from society and relationships, of course." **Student**

"Myself." **Student**

"Intrinsic motivation. I have my own goals." **Student**

I was surprised to learn that most of the students still ate some sort of breakfast, most of the time, some sort of lunch, generally speaking, and seldom ate high-fat, fast food. When I asked if they worried about getting fat, of the ones who answered, 10 girls said yes and three said no, five boys said yes and four said no. I wanted to know how they felt the media influenced their self-perception.

"I never think of myself as perfect because of the media. There is always something 'wrong' with me according to media stereotypes. I know that is wrong yet I still believe it. I want perfect curves and to be skinny, yet that is nearly impossible. However, it is what is expected of me, according to the media." **Student**

"The media makes you think that being skinny makes you sexy and wanted and that anyone with a little bit of fat is ugly and overweight." **Student**

"The media affects the way I look at my body. It makes me want to be skinnier in order to be accepted by society." **Student**

"The media is a distortion of lies so I don't pay attention to it." **Student**

"I put myself down a lot. I don't think I'm pretty or have a good body, and most of that comes from a stereotypical image of what the media says you're supposed to look like." **Student**

"It makes me feel unattractive and overweight at times." **Student**

"It makes girls feel like they need to be skinny and attractive to be liked." **Student**

"I realize that the media uses tactics to attack teenagers' insecurities." **Student**

"The media makes me think about how glad I am that I'm not fat!" **Student**

This age group was open, respectful, charismatic, entertaining, and motivated. What I found most interesting came at the end of the session when I asked the students what they looked for in the opposite sex. The girls had 12 characteristics before the guys finished digesting the question, then they started with looks, although it is hard to say if they were just kidding. The girls listed, in no particular order, sense of humor, height, personal hygiene, athletic ability, personality, maturity, muscles, nice teeth, being well-dressed, confidence, sensitivity, non-smoking, non-drug-using, respectful towards others, and making a good first impression. Nothing about looks or body size. The guys said, in no particular order, looks, personality, intelligence, teeth, eyes, legs, athleticism, confidence, security, non-smoking, non-promiscuous, not ditsy, and a healthy weight. When I asked them what a "healthy" weight meant, they all agreed that girls think guys are attracted to skinny but guys are attracted to a "healthy" weight—curves and breasts. "Interesting," I thought.

Times change.

As a teenager I can remember, quite vividly, the stresses of growing up and trying to become independent with limited tools and a big ego. Moving nine times by Grade 9 and the daughter of the chief of police just made me that much more headstrong and independent. I thought I could do everything on my own, with no help from anyone. If I was told to do something by an adult, they had better be prepared to give me a plausible reason why, because I always figured I deserved an explanation, much to my parents' nervousness. The day after I graduated I hopped on a Greyhound bus with my 25 pairs of jeans and 12 pairs of Nike runners I had worked so hard for, and left Alberta, bound for British Columbia to visit my best friend. It never dawned on me that this might be dangerous. Hell, I was 17—pretty much invincible. Several hundred miles and several weeks later, I landed in Kelowna, BC with a few hundred dollars in my bank account and big ambitions. Get out of my way—I was like a steam train rolling with no apparent brakes. Mom always said, "If there is a brick wall, Mia will go through it, not over it."

I didn't worry about crystal meth, E (ecstasy), depression, AIDS, HIV, rape, or date-rape. I didn't worry about kidnapping or robbery, drinking and driving, getting fat, wearing a helmet, wearing a seat belt, or wearing sunscreen. I didn't worry about Internet porn, cyber bullying, the bird flu, greenhouse emissions, nuclear war or cancer. I didn't worry about not getting a job, where I would live, how I would live or what would happen if I needed help. Those things would just happen. I lived in an exciting, adventurous, happy, safe world of sunshine, cute guys, coolers, aerobics classes, downhill skiing and freedom.

Today young girls and boys live in a very different world. They live in a world of extreme social pressures ranging from dangerous sex and drugs to the ultra-thin epidemic. They are bombarded with messages intent on luring them into believing what they need, what they should look like, and how they should act. The incidence of sexual abuse, depression, chronic diseases, and eating disorders is beyond the scope of our understanding. The idea of a young adult in today's inflated society, being able to live on their own, working one full-time job is not possible. It takes two or three student incomes to be able to afford rent, not to mention all the other things that society has made them believe they need, such as cell phones, pagers, cable television, plasma screens, MSN, computers, new cars, and fancy brand name clothes. It's no wonder young adults eat the way they do. There is no money left over for healthy food choices. Kraft Dinner and Ichiban have become a fifth food group.

The more advanced technology becomes, the more violent the media becomes, the more disposable society becomes, the greater the divide between the rich and the poor becomes, the more people prey on other people's weaknesses, the more dangerous our world will become.

As long as we live in this world we will not be able to stop progress and change but we can adjust the way we choose to participate in it.

As I write this book, Hilary Clinton is preparing her campaign for the Presidency of the United States. Angelina Jolie is creating more awareness of the hardships in Third World countries, since Princess Diana. Oprah Winfrey is single-handedly removing pedophiles from the back alleys of our communities, one pedophile at a time. The list goes on and on. Take a look at what women are accomplishing in your community. Young women of this generation have the opportunity to facilitate the greatest positive changes in the world through education, motivation, determination, access and strength in numbers, but they can't do it if all they can think about is how fat they look in their jeans.

Take your daughters by the hand and lead them away from the caustic influences of their generation. Show them that they can be and can do anything. Make them believe that size doesn't matter, health does. Join them in a fitness class. Take them on an adventure. Volunteer with them. Teach them how to read a book for entertainment. Shut the television off. Limit computer time. Stop complaining about your weight. Take the focus off hair, make-up and clothes. Put the emphasis on moving, exploring, learning and growing. Discipline them. Put boundaries on them. Nurture them. Nourish them. Love them. Tall, short, fat, skinny, blue eyes, brown eyes, big boobs, little boobs, blonde hair, red hair, freckles, zits, curly hair—it doesn't matter. The shell that these little girls come in has nothing to do with what they have the potential to accomplish.

9
EXERCISE

"I just make the best of my body while the aging process continues. I try to keep in the best shape I can. The reward is looking the best I can at that particular point in my life. It is an ever-changing, dynamic process."

Interview client #53

"If my clothes fit, it is all good but what is more important to my happiness is exercise. If I am moving my body then I have an overall sense of happiness with my weight and my emotional state." **Interview client #57**

"Being thin doesn't equal happiness per se but being fit does."

Interview client #42

"Everyday I feel lucky to have a healthy body with which to enjoy my life." **Interview client #36**

"To be truthful I never weigh myself because it is just a number and I figure if you eat well and get the right amount of exercise then it shouldn't matter what you weigh."

Interview client #63

"When I feel good about myself I am happy. If I am feeling fit and strong I feel together and that I can do anything. It's not very often I don't feel good about myself these days."

Interview client #40

"I am happiest when I feel good about how I look. Strong and lean make me happy." **Interview client #36**

"Weight has never been linked to happiness for me. For me, the higher the number is on the scale, the more muscle I have. As soon as that number drops I know I am slacking on the weights." **Interview client #32**

For any of you who have joined a gym or are currently a member at a gym, can you identify with the following? The trainer takes you through an orientation and shows you how to use the treadmill or the bike. She sets the machine for 20 minutes, using the manual program and suggests that you keep your heart rate in a certain range for optimal benefits. Before she is out of sight, you shut the treadmill down and re-start the machine using the *fat burn* program! Most commercial pieces of cardio equipment have the *fat burn* program built in. This program is meant to control the speed of the cardio equipment based on your heart rate, your age and the appropriate exercise zone. If your heart rate is too high for your age the machine will automatically slow down and if your heart rate is too low for your age, it will automatically speed up. What people actually think when they push the *fat burn* button is that the machine will suck all the fat out of their legs by the end of the 20 minute workout or they will receive a full refund on their gym membership. If the button said *salad burn*, it would never get pushed.

Having owned a fitness centre for nine years and worked in them for 20 years, I've had the opportunity to witness some pretty interesting methods of weight reduction. Love the fat reduction suits designed to increase your internal core temperature to that of the Sahara Desert at noon, in order to burn more calories. What about the fat jiggler machine. Fabulous! Stand on the machine, wrap the belt around your butt and thighs and jiggle your way to thinness—no caloric expenditure required. The muscle stimulation machines designed to burn as many calories in 20 minutes as an aerobics class. Then there are the 'Fat Burn', 'Butt Buster', 'Gut Buster', 'Long and Lean' classes that simply by attending, you're guaranteed results because of the name of the class. What about cellulite creams that burn off stored fat. Ahhahahahhaa!

I've watched members work out at 6 a.m. come back at 9 a.m. and then just for good measure, one more workout after school. I wanted to eat just watching them. Try wearing the fat reduction suit on the treadmill while pumping to Michael Jackson and wearing ankle weights. No? How about sets of 100 reps or no less than 50 sets of exercises per workout. Sound ridiculous? It is!

Small victories lead to big victories. Five pounds each month, 60 pounds by the end of the year. Three *sensible* one-hour workouts a week, 156 hours of exercise by the end of the year—approximately 62,000 calories expended (based on 400 calories an hour), by years end. Cut out sweets six days a week, reduce your caloric intake by thousands by the end of the year. I didn't say eliminate and I didn't say every day!

Exercise is a gift! Many of you may think I should take a walk to the closest hospital and admit myself but I believe that to be a fact. If you were crippled, a quadriplegic, a severe diabetic, had horrible rheumatoid arthritis, suffered from fibromyalgia or chronic fatigue and couldn't exercise, you would realize how badly you wished you could swim or walk or run or do yoga or hike or bike or whatever your exercise of choice is. Because many of us are not faced with potentially debilitating conditions, we take our body and we take exercise for granted. It will be there tomorrow, nibble, nibble, nibble. We can do something about it tomorrow, nibble, nibble, nibble. I'll join a gym tomorrow, nibble, nibble, nibble. I don't have time to exercise, nibble, nibble, nibble.

Having owned a gym for years, I will be the first one to tell you *not* to join a gym unless that is what you truly love to do for exercise. I told people that when we owned Fitness Excellence and I tell you that now. Not everyone is a gym rat. Thinking if you buy into a long term contract, you'll guilt yourself into going? Doesn't work that way. The gym owner loves this type of client. They don't produce any wear and tear on the equipment. After three weeks they quit going but their money continues to pay the facility owner's mortgage. Do what you truly love to do and you know you will incorporate into your life—for life.

When someone asks me, "What is the *best* exercise I can do for weight loss and health", I tell them that cross-country skiing is by far the best overall, low-impact, calorie burning activity. So what if you live in Las Vegas or Puerto Vallarta or San Diego or Cairo? Does that mean, "Thank God I don't have to exercise because the *best* exercise isn't available to me"? No, what it means is that the best exercise for you is that which you love to do and will include in your life, for life. Walk, hike, bike, swim, dance, golf, yoga, belly dance, bowl, bird watch, whatever you love to do. If you don't like any form of exercise, and there are lots of people out there who don't, simply pick the simplest and most accessible form of exercise that doesn't require you to buy a bunch of expensive equipment or sign in blood. A great choice is walking.

Weight loss without exercise is not fat loss.

When people begin to understand and accept that one of the essential elements of successful weight loss and weight management is exercise, they will be on the road to success. If you are reading this book right now, you can no longer use the excuses, "I don't have time or I can't afford it". If you are reading this book, you have both the time and the money to exercise! Walking only costs a pair of shoes. Dancing in your home only takes turning on the radio. Pushing your child in their stroller to the store only takes a stroller. Buying a used treadmill out of the newspaper just takes a bit of time and money. Bird watching only takes a notebook and a some sunscreen. Think about all the money you have spent on diet gimmicks that didn't work. Now take that same amount of money, desire and time and start spending it on your health.

You *will not* and *cannot* lose weight or maintain weight without exercise. Accept it now. Choose what you are going to include in your life and go for it. Set a great example for your children. If your child is watching Sesame Street, hop on your treadmill and watch it with them. Start playing soccer or basketball or catch with your children after school. Who cares if you are no good at it. Do you think your kids care? All they care about is that they are playing and you are playing with them. Go swimming. Can't image being caught dead in a bathing suit? Well dead is going to be the way your body feels after

20 or 30 years of not exercising. Ride your bike with them. What a great excuse to get a funky new outfit! Walk up and down your stairs 10 times before the kids get up, 10 more times after you drop them off at school, 10 more times before you eat dinner and 10 more times before you pick the kids up. You get the picture. Have you ever heard that clever line, 'Dance like no one is watching'? Put on your favorite CD and make a fool out of yourself for half an hour. Who knows, you may become a better dancer!

Avoid believing the key to weight loss is the next fad diet and start to acknowledge that exercise is one of the key components to weight loss. Any weight loss program without exercise is just another get rich gimmick that is bound to fail and make you feel like a failure.

Set a goal and learn to love the journey. Goals come in all sizes, shapes and desires. Regardless of your desire, whether it is to be rich, to move, to have another child, to go on a vacation or to lose weight, you have to have a goal and you have to break the goal down into manageable steps that will lead to your success. Next, establish a timeframe or a deadline. Without deadlines, your goals are just dreams. It is easy to say I want to be healthy or I want to lose weight or I want to be skinny, but none of those goals are tangible. How about I want to reduce my blood pressure by five percent within two months? That is a tangible way of saying I want to be healthy. How about I want to lose 10 pounds by June? That is a tangible way of saying I want to lose weight. How about I want to go from a size 16 to a size 12 by summer? That is a tangible way of saying I want to be skinny. Once you have established a tangible goal, sit down and figure out what lifestyle changes are going to be necessary to attain your goal. Create a very detailed plan, with baby steps, because willpower won't work. For example, I am no longer going to eat French fries, I am going to walk for 25 minutes every day after I drop the kids off at school, whenever I feel like grazing out of boredom I am going to take a bath, I'm going to include two vegetables with each supper. Forget about the expectation and focus on the progress.

Lastly, make yourself accountable to someone! Regardless of who, find someone that is going to watch and celebrate your victories with you. Someone that can motivate you when you are feeling weak or tired. Someone that inspires you to keep moving toward your goal. Someone that understands and loves you. It may be a person or it may be a support group. You are your motivator but they are your conscience.

"Don't focus on the outcome, focus on the journey."
Interview client #64

"It will take time but I will do it and it will be because of life-style changes." **Interview client #60**

"Workout with another person. It is harder to let someone else down than it is yourself." **Interview client #51**

"Don't ever give up! Even though you think you can't get to where you want to be, you can, you just have to make a goal."
Interview client #37

Start living the life you dream of.

Once you have established your goal, determined the steps required to attain your goal and selected someone to be accountable to, sit back and enjoy the journey. Enjoy the process of change. Nothing will change until you make it happen. Enjoy every step of every day as you move closer and closer to your goal and off this desperate journey. Don't be afraid of saying goodbye to the old lifestyle, the old friends and the old you! Don't be afraid of setbacks and don't be afraid of change. Many of the women that I talked to expressed a dislike and a fear of change. If you think about it rationally, change is one of the few things that is constant in life. Everything is constantly changing. The weather, our age, our children's age, our appearance, our perceptions, our communities, our likes, our mates, our homes, our shoes, our pets, our schools, and so on and so on and so on. Stop and think about change as an opportunity for growth rather than a hurdle that paralyzes you. This will only keep you from setting and reaching your goals. Imagine if Rick Hansen, Oprah Winfrey, Terry Fox, Mother Teresa and Lady Diana didn't think about change as an opportunity for a better world.

"I wanted permanent, healthy weight loss so bad that I was willing to change my life for it." **Interview client #60**

Exercise for many people is a change they are petrified of. They are petrified of failing, of feeling discomfort, of sweating, of making a fool out of themselves, of hurting themselves. Take a look at each one of these examples and ask yourself if failing at something is better or worse than having never tried. How could someone possibly fail at exercise, other than to join an activity and not participate in it. The only way you can fail at exercise is by never attempting it. Feeling discomfort. What is worse, the feeling of being 60 pounds overweight, hating yourself and your body and being a slave to food or a bit of sweat running down the crack of your butt when you're out for a walk? Sweating! I bet that happens when you have sex or are sitting on the beach in Hawaii and you probably don't mind it then. Sweating is one of the cheapest ways to rid the body of toxins, so enjoy it— it's a free detox. Making a fool out of yourself. Ah, this one I hear all the time. I hear people say they couldn't possibly join a gym because everyone would stare at them. I always think this is a rather self-centered statement to make. Hate to burst your excuse bubble but no one cares who you are or what you look like, they are all there for the same reason and that is to improve their health. Lastly, is the I might hurt myself excuse. Please believe that you are going to hurt yourself far worse if you don't start to exercise. You're going to increase your chances of heart disease, cancer, diabetes, tendonitis, arthritis, osteoporosis and obesity, not to mention mental anguish.

I want you to write down every excuse you use to keep from exercising, starting with the, "I don't have time" one, keeping in mind that you have the same number of hours in a day as Rick Hansen, Lance Armstrong, Mother Teresa, Terry Fox and Martin Luther King. Do you watch television? Are you reading this book? Do you watch your children when they play? Do you spend time having coffee with your girlfriends? Do you go to bed late and wake up when you absolutely have to and no sooner? Do you sit in the lunch room at lunch time after having sat all morning at your desk job? Do you have the energy to shop? Do you have the money for a Starbucks coffee every morning? Do you eat out two or three times a week? Then you have the time and the money to exercise. Have you used any or all of the excuses I have listed and more? Then you are out of excuses! Thomas Fuller once said, "Bad excuses are worse than none".

Fit and fat?

Did you know that you can be fit and be fat? Some of the fittest people I have known and taught, were fat. One of the best fitness classes I ever participated in was taught by a set of fat sisters, and I mean really fat. One of my favorite programs that I had the pleasure of teaching was a program called Fitness Plus. The prerequisite was that you had to be fat to participate. I am five foot seven, 120 pounds and am a respectable athlete but I have been passed in run races by women 30 pounds heavier than me. I say, "Good on you". I participated in a 15km power walk with one of my clients, who at the time was 25 pounds overweight. She had already lost 50 pounds and would end up losing 100 pounds in one year. I am trying to say that sometimes, heavy does not mean unfit or unhealthy, just like skinny does not mean fit and healthy.

I read a very interesting article about a man named David Alexander. He is the co-owner of an oil company in Phoenix, Arizona and he is a fat triathlete. He is five foot eight and weighs 250 pounds. Considered obese because of his height and weight, his body and his mind have completed over 270 triathlons in 37 countries. For those of you who are not familiar with a triathlon, it is a race where the athlete swims 2.4 miles, bikes 112 miles and then runs a marathon. Alexander also completed an ultra distance triathlon consisting of a 9.6 mile swim, a 448 mile ride and a 104.8 mile run in 85 hours, 46 minutes and 38 seconds. The article was called, *The Fittest Fat Man*. Imagine being passed by him.

We need to change our perceptions and open our minds to the possibility that fit and healthy can come in a multitude of sizes and shapes. Fit and healthy is not reflected on the catwalks of New York, it is reflected on the sidewalks of our communities. It is a reflection of the 60-year-old woman on the hiking trails of the Grand Canyon, the fitness centers of our communities, the aquatic classes at our pools, the 6 a.m. runs in the pouring rain and the dragon boating sessions on Thursday nights. It is not reflected in the size of your jeans, the size of your bra, the style of your underwear or the number on the scale.

Every time you embark on another diet, you sell your soul to the Diet God and make the diet industry a little richer. The more women fail at dieting, the more successful the diet industry becomes. We have never heard the weight loss industry referred to as the fat loss industry because what you lose has little to do with fat. How ironic. Everyone is trying so hard to be skinny but the diet industry is designed to make you a fat skinny person. When you weigh yourself every Friday morning, naked, before breakfast, coffee or water and the scale tells you that you lost three pounds this week, you're elated. What it doesn't tell you is what you lost. Did you lose a bowel movement or two, a couple of litres of water and a few more brain cells? Chances are pretty good that what you lost has little to do with fat, especially if the diet is a low calorie diet designed to test your human fortitude and your will to live. By the end of the diet, you have lost 25 pounds in six weeks. On a diet plan such as this, the majority of what you will lose will be water and muscle, which actually makes you fatter than you were when you started, even though the scale tells you what you want to see. Would you rather be a fat skinny person or a fit fat person? Would you rather prescribe to the healthy pill or the skinny pill? Would you rather be 150 pounds and 25 per cent body fat or 120 pounds and 32 per cent body fat?

"My well-being, physically and emotionally, is due to a good exercise program and sensible eating."
                                        Interview client #36

"My weight isn't an issue, but my health is."
                                        Interview client #24

"I like my body even though it is not perfect. I now look at the fat I carry as my 'future energy stores'. If I start to feel unhappy about it I focus on eating healthy and eating to have energy." **Interview client #35**

I turned 40 and I was fat!

I've heard so many women use this line, except the age isn't always the same. I turned 25 and boom—I was fat. They said when you turn 30 your body changes. When you turn 40 your body sags. I would like to chronicle someone's life from their 29th birthday to their 30th birthday and see if they wake up fat between the last night of their 29th year and the first morning of their 30th year. Women will say it with that much conviction.

Let's look at it a bit more realistically. When you graduate from high school, you weigh 120 pounds (in your dreams some of you are saying). Okay, how about 140 pounds? You go to university and you gain the required 20 'study' pounds by the time you graduate four years later (if you didn't party year one away). That is only five pounds a year. Now you weigh 160 pounds and you carry it pretty well. You meet Prince Charming, have a whirlwind couple of years before settling down to have kids. You manage to avoid gaining any more weight. You get a job, have two kids and gain six pounds a year for the next four years. You wake up on your 30th birthday weighing 184 pounds. Five pounds more a year and you wake up on your 40th birthday and you weigh 234 pounds, 94 pounds more than you did when you graduated. Just in time for your high school reunion. Not a chance you say. I turned 40 and I was fat!

Weight gain can be very insidious if you aren't paying attention. It's like grey hair, wrinkles, balding, and poor posture.

It happens so gradually that we have plenty of time to get used to the look and feeling. We may not like it but we don't really notice how gradually it is happening. If we think about gaining three pounds a year, it really isn't much. That is only an additional 10,500 stored fat calories or .13151 of an ounce per day or an additional 28 calories a day either consumed or not burned off. Very insidious, very subtle, very manageable and downright sneaky. You wake up on your 40th birthday, 69 pounds heavier than you were when you graduated.

Sadly, most women would wish it was only three pounds a year. Imagine *only* gaining eight pounds a year—184 pounds when you turn 40. Couple this overwhelming figure with a sedentary lifestyle, loss of muscle mass, a depressed metabolism, poor nutritional habits, a lengthy history of dieting and poor family genetics and you have managed to establish a perfect fat storing environment. Your fat cells are celebrating and the buffet is you!

Be accountable, take responsibility and commit to change —for life. Don't get depressed and pull the kitchen chair up to the fridge—get focused. What is done is done. Just like you managed to gain 184 pounds or 100 pounds or 60 pounds, you can lose it too. Just remember, if it took you 20 years to put it on, don't expect to lose it in 10 weeks regardless of what the North Beach/Zoned Out/Akne/Slam Fist/L.A. Wait Lost/Nutra-ridiculous System say. Do it the right way with lifestyle changes, commitment, patience, motivation, and accountability. Accept responsibility, outline your goals, believe in yourself and go for it one day, one meal and one function at a time.

The fitness bank

Every time you exercise think about it as making a deposit

into your fitness bank. Over time, all those deposits accrue interest and that interest is health and longevity. On the other hand, when you go away on holidays or just don't feel like exercising one day, think of it as a withdrawal. Over time, all that matters is that you make more deposits than you do withdrawals.

When I go on holidays, sometimes the opportunity for me to enjoy the amount of exercise or the type of exercise that I would typically participate in, may not be realistic. My exercise regime gets turned upside down and I just have to remember that I have made enough deposits over the past several months that I can live off the interest and not have to worry. I might not feel as great and I may gain a pound or two but the overall picture is what is most important.

10
CONSEQUENCES

"She refused to admit that she had a problem, and told us that she was growing up and that her metabolism was changing. She was a dancer from the age of five, and dance was her passion. Eventually she danced with a semi-professional dance group, which continued for one or two years. When she was in Grade 2 a substitute teacher was doing comparisons. She pointed to a boy in the class, saying that he was the *skinny* one and then pointed to our daughter and said she was the *fat* one—which she wasn't, she was just a solid little girl, absolutely not fat. In high school, during puberty, she did put on some weight. She was a beautiful and talented dancer, and her success in making it into the semi-professional dance group was ridiculed by some of her close peers, who were jealous of her success. Nasty notes were left in her locker, and I know she turned to school counselors and dance teachers with her pain of this ridicule. Her weight slowly started to drop in Grade 12, and now at the age of 20, she is 96 pounds."

Mother

Let's talk about the consequences that constant dieting and dysfunctional eating habits have on our body image. Let's talk about the consequences of dieting, dysfunctional eating and poor body-image on our children, more specifically our daughters. The trauma we cause ourselves, our friends and our families can be as devastating as the physical consequences of an eating disorder, with one major difference. The physical trauma we do to ourselves, the mental and emotional trauma we do to ourselves as well as our friends and our families. Listening to so many women talk about dysfunctional eating, I have come to realize that constant dieting not only has a lasting effect on ourselves but also on the ones we love.

The consequences are as dangerous emotionally as they are physically. We are dieting ourselves to fatness. We are dieting ourselves to diabetes. We are dieting ourselves to depression. We are dieting ourselves to obesity. We are dieting ourselves to divorce. We are dieting ourselves to suicide. We are dieting ourselves to liposuction and gastric bypass surgery. We are dieting our daughters to fatness, diabetes, depression, obesity, divorce, liposuction and gastric bypass surgery, and suicide. We are dieting our daughter's daughters to fatness, diabetes, depression, obesity, divorce, liposuction and gastric bypass surgery and suicide. We are doing it to ourselves and we are doing it to our daughters and they are doing it to their daughters. The cycle needs to be broken and it can be broken if we stop handing our dysfunctional relationship with food down to our daughters.

Our addiction to thin has made food the most widely abused substance in society. We don't take the time to think about the consequences of what it takes to become thin, we only think about the concept of thin. In the process of groping and frantically clawing our way to thinness, we lose living along the way.

We lose life, love, relationships and happiness.

"I turned down life experiences and opportunities that were presented to me. Because I thought I was too fat. I didn't pursue them. My girlfriends just went to Hawaii for a week and invited me but the thought of wearing a bathing suit kept me from going. My girlfriends would be so upset if they knew that was the reason."　**Interview client #20**
(10 pounds overweight)

"All of my dieting has made me lose control over my life."
Interview client #14

"I lost a whole entire part of myself that I don't have any idea how to get back. The part of me that I lost is the part of me that used to know what it was like to feel good about myself. To wake up in the morning with no thoughts of food or what people think I look like. I lost who I truly am."
Interview client #15

"I have lost so many missed opportunities and memories that I could have had, by either being preoccupied with my disorder or by not feeling good about what I looked like or by not feeling good and not participating in things."
Interview client #13

"I have lost myself. Mostly from feeling bad about my appearance. I have stayed away from situations, from people, and from doing things that I would have liked."
Interview client #60

"Because of dieting, I have lost my self-esteem."
Interview client #51

"I lost who I was when I lost all that weight."
Interview client #11

"I lost 15 years of my life and my dream of becoming a writer because of my obsession with thin."
Interview client #12

"I lost friends because I didn't keep in touch with them as they moved away. As I gained weight, I didn't want them to see me this big." **Interview client #61**

Each time we make a conscious or unconscious decision to not eat or to self-loathe or to yell at our children because we are angry at our self or to sit in front of the television for hours on end, we send a message to our children. When that behavior is repeated over and over again, it becomes a learned trait. Our children begin to think not eating is acceptable, self-loathing is normal, yelling is a standard method of communication and watching television for hours is brain exercise. We either have to accept the consequences of our actions or change our actions. Newton's Law states—*For every action, there is an equal and opposite reaction.*

Consequences are the effect, result or outcome of an action. If the consequence of constant yo-yo dieting is fatness and self-loathing then why participate? If dieting makes you miserable and makes your family miserable then why play the game? If you can't find a diet that works maybe it's because they don't. If not exercising compromises your quality of life, why not get up and move? If your weight causes you to worry about your health and your future, start doing something about it. If the current diet that you are on gives you headaches, mood swings, cravings and makes you irritable, then throw it on the pile with the other diets and walk away. Enjoy the consequences of your actions instead of denying yourself the right to happiness and contentment. It is inevitable that dieting will fail to bring you the results you are looking for. It is inevitable that making changes *to your* diet will bring you positive lasting results. It is a fact that you will not lose the type of weight you want through restricted caloric programs. It is a fact that you will lose body fat if you begin to include exercise in your daily routine. You will always chase the elusive number on the weigh scale as long as you continue to diet. If you make positive changes to your diet and your lifestyle it will eventually be reflected by the number on the scale. Continuing to eat foods that are high in sugar and additives will continue to promote uncontrollable mood swings. Decreasing the amount of processed foods in your diet will help stabilize your blood sugar and even out your temperament. Get off the diet treadmill and you will start to live. Action—consequence. Positive—negative. You control the outcome.

"It is very difficult as I have been like this for longer than I can remember. It is part of who I am. I don't know how to be any other way."   **Interview client #42**

"For me this journey will never end although a number on the scale will finish one chapter."   **Interview client #61**

"My body makes me sad, I wish it was better. I wish I could find a boyfriend to love me."   **Grade 6 student**

"If you think you're just kind of not okay now, you'll hate yourself by the time this dieting game ends."
                                                      Interview client #46

"I don't like my body and I wish I was someone else."
                                                         Grade 7 student

"When you are so unhappy and you hit rock bottom, you come to a point when you are prepared to do anything. This is not living. You must want it badly enough to change."

Interview client #12

Typical consequences of dysfunctional eating and eating disorders.

- erosion of the stomach lining
- acid reflux disorders
- electrolyte imbalances
- hair loss
- digestive difficulties
- noticeably unhealthy skin, hair and nails
- diabetes
- gum disease
- loss of tooth enamel
- tooth loss
- depression
- TMJ (issues with the jaw locking from repeated bouts of purging)
- dehydration
- issues with bowel movements and urinary problems
- peptic ulcers
- callused fingers from repeated bouts of self induced vomiting - (Russell's sign)
- swelling of the face from purging and dehydration
- tearing of the esophagus
- weakness from loss of muscle and lack of food
- issues with low blood pressure constantly making the person dizzy and light headed
- soft downy hair on the face and body to help keep the body warm
- drug abuse

- lack of self-respect
- sadness
- low self-esteem
- chronic fatigue
- seizures
- esophageal cancer
- amenorrhea (loss of menstruation)
- insomnia
- infertility
- anemia (low iron levels)
- kidney failure
- heart failure
- liver failure
- atrophy (muscle loss)
- osteoporosis
- pancreatitis
- loneliness
- loss of relationships
- suicide
- fear
- DEATH

Being thin is it!

Payback

Our body can hold a grudge longer than the high school girl whose boyfriend you married. It can hold the consequences of our actions against us for life, but it can also provide us with amazing gifts such as childbirth and breast feeding.

For most people, what we do to our body is accumulative. If we choose to not brush our teeth, it is likely that we will one day suffer from tooth decay. If we lead a sedentary life, there is a very good chance that one day we will suffer from heart disease, lack of mobility, and weight issues. If we choose to eat primarily processed food, chances are we will suffer from obesity, cancer, and chronic fatigue. If we choose to wear high heels everyday, we are likely to end up with short heel chords, bunions and low back pain. If, however, we choose to exercise three to five times per week and eat a healthy, balanced diet, chances are we are going to enjoy a higher quality of life. Chances are we will decrease our risk of heart disease, of being overweight, of certain types of cancer, of diabetes, of osteoporosis as well as decrease our chance of depression, anger, resentment, sadness and fear.

What we do to our body and what we put into our body is a collective journey. We may not see the effects today or tomorrow but eventually the effects are going to show up. Everybody gets the body they deserve—eventually. This is true for positive outcomes such as being fit and healthy or negative outcomes such as weight gain, diabetes and depression. Don't get deluded in the belief that you have gotten away with an unhealthy approach to eating for this long, so you will get away with it forever.

What we have done in the past has gotten us to where we are in the present and what we do in the present determines where we will be in the future. The three are intertwined like pieces of a puzzle. This goes for many aspects of our life. Yesterday, today and tomorrow. Learn from the past, enjoy the present, look forward to the future.

Blaming

When we begin to realize that we are ultimately responsible for ourselves and that blaming is just a way of prolonging what we don't want to accept, the sooner we will be able to take our destiny into our hands. Women either need to learn to accept their weight, if they are not willing to make the appropriate lifestyle changes, or they need to stop complaining, get uncomfortable with the process and enjoy the results.

Alcoholics Anonymous defines insanity as—*continuing the same behavior and expecting a different result*. The dictionary defines insanity as extremely foolish and hare-brained. Every diet a woman embarks on is the same behavior with the hopes of a different result. A different spin on insanity. A different spin on when to eat, how much to eat, how to eat, who to eat with, where to eat, what color the food should be, what shape the veggies should be, what music to listen to in order to aid in digestion and how to create flat abs while you eat. All with the same outcome or consequence—failure. Let's be clear, I'm not talking diabetic diets or *Weight Watchers* or medically prescribed diets; you all know which ones I am talking about. The ones that tell you not to eat unless it is out of their can, box, book or bag with the name of the wizard who invented it— along with the special motivational DVD that is yours for 37 per cent less, if you purchase today—plus you'll also receive the bonus fat gobbler pills. Those diets!

When the diet fails, don't blame the diet, don't blame the weather, don't blame your kids or your husband, and don't blame your genetics, accept the blame. You made the decision to buy into the gimmick, therefore you must accept the consequences.

It sounds very insensitive and callous, but you know what you have to do to lose weight and it doesn't come from another diet book or another diet program. It comes from stopping the old habits and replacing them with positive lifestyle changes.

The next time someone tells you about the fabulous Eskimo diet they are on, as much as you are going to want to go out and buy the dehydrated whale blubber and the fat metabolizing seal cream, smile and politely decline. Tell them you have found the diet that works. It is going to take time, dedication, perseverance and patience but eventually the outcome will be worth the work. Consequences—that which naturally follows from preceding actions.

"Throughout this process I have learned that I am responsible for everything in my life." **Interview client #43**

11
HOPE

To desire with the expectation of fulfillment. Hope is the carrot that eternally bobs out in front of our nose. It is the mirage in the desert. It is our lifeline to happiness. Without hope there can be death. For people who were stuck in the rubble of the Twin Towers or wedged in a tree with a broken pelvis during the tsunami in Thailand, or lying on top of the roof of their house with two dogs and three scared children after Hurricane Katrina left the husband dead, or in Africa watching while his wife and three children are murdered—sometimes the only thing that keeps people alive is hope. In the media recently, young Shawn Hornbeck, who was kidnapped by Michael Devlin at the age of 11 and rescued at the age of 15, said the only thing that kept him going was the *hope* that he would one day be found and reunited with his parents.

We hope for a better life. We hope our children stay safe. We hope we can pay the bills next month. We hope this damn diet will work. We hope our husband still finds us attractive.

We hope our basement doesn't flood. We hope we can lose 10 pounds for our sister's wedding. We hope, we hope, we hope.

Hope doesn't transpire just because we desire it to happen. I hope my son lives a long, healthy, happy life and I do everything in my power to ensure his health and happiness while I can. I hope that I can make life a little easier for people and I am attempting to do that through this book. I hope I lead a long, healthy life and I work very hard at my lifestyle to improve those chances. Hope takes work, hope takes commitment, hope takes change, hope takes time. Weight loss takes work, weight loss takes commitment, weight loss takes change, weight loss takes time. I didn't say Die with a t, I said weight loss because you can hope a diet will work all you want, but diet is not the key to weight loss; work, commitment, lifestyle changes, time, and patience along with the physiological components we previously talked about, are the key.

When we lose faith in the hope that we will one day be slimmer, we begin the journey down the road to obesity. When we lose faith in the hope we can no longer control food, we become caught in the grip of eating disorders. Hope is sometimes all that sets us apart from the homeless person on the street or the lady next door that weighs 550 pounds. I received a brilliant e-mail from one of the women I interviewed and it made me smile from my heart when I read it because it is what I *hope* for women struggling with this journey.

"One of the biggest steps in my recovery was simply making a clear decision that I was ready to learn to eat like a normal person (ie. a person without an eating disorder). After all the hows and whys of spending so much of my life with bulimia and being a slave to eating and food, I realized that I was the only one in control of why, when and what I put in my body. As

I started coming out of my depression, my thinking about my relationship with food started changing as well. I began to watch how other people ate, and discovered that (to my surprise!) most people ate because they were hungry and stopped eating when they had had enough! I quietly observed people and how they behaved around food, friends, family and strangers. I discovered that many people without eating disorders occasionally would overeat at family gatherings, holidays, etc. but the difference between how they managed their overeating and how I did was a real learning experience for me. First of all, it made me realize that overeating from time to time didn't mean one had an eating disorder, just that nearly everyone likes to indulge once in a while. I saw that normal eaters didn't feel guilty about overeating, and still had their limits (unlike my solitary binges). Also, people quite openly would eat a little more than they needed, sometimes even a lot more, and not be ashamed of it, even laugh and joke about it. I discovered that often when people overate, they would compensate for it the next day by eating small amounts—in other words, they would listen to their body! This was a foreign concept to me. It was like learning how to eat normally, a step I guess I missed out on when I was growing up. I started to try and copy the eating behaviors of normal eaters—my theory being that of simple behavior modification (of course, it wasn't simple, it took a lot of determination and strength). I still find myself observing how others eat—how some people attach so much emotional energy to food and eating, how others simply eat for fuel and don't seem to care much about what they eat (mostly men), how some are mostly concerned about eating healthy foods but not concerned about calories, and how a few people seem to have no interest at all in food and eating, and really have to have meals prepared for them in order to eat nutritiously (again, mainly men). I continue in this recovery mode—but feel enlightened since our interview. I binged and purged the evening after our interview, then started to feel angry at myself for this, but managed to turn it around into an opportunity for change. I made a fresh decision not to purge again—to put that behavior in the past." *Hope.* **Interview client #38**

If you can raise healthy, mentally stable children, you can find peace with your body. If you can obtain a PhD, you can find peace with your body. If you can juggle a career, a husband, a family, you can find peace with your body. If you realize you need to heal the past and learn to love yourself then there is hope—hope for a better today which will become a better tomorrow.

Let's start a diet revolution!

Let's stand up, as a wonderful, wise and competent sector of society, and say, "We are not going to listen to your bullshit anymore! We don't care what you deem as acceptable. I am acceptable. We will not throw our money away to the diet industry any longer. We will take that money and spend it on us. We will tell the grocery stores to stick their fashion magazines right next to Fly Fishing and Horse Quarterly, if not, perhaps somewhere a bit more humbling. We will look at television shows that exploit women through fake hair, fake boobs, fake teeth, fake, fake, fake, and say, 'No thanks, I'll watch something a bit more intelligent.' We will tell the people in our life that judge us based on our external appearance, 'Smell ya later dude.' We will stop buying fat trappers, metabolic enhancers, fat melting creams, eyelid hooks, chin bras, tricep slings, corsets, breakfast in a can, 12 steps to a rock-hard butt, 30 minutes to perfection, the 4 minute workout, the 7 minute workout, the workout with no sweat, fat jigglers, fat zappers, fat suckers, compression suits, push up bras (well, maybe we shouldn't get too hasty), cellulite creams (come on gals!), power suits designed to detox your liver, muscle stimulation machines, Phen/ fen, chromium picolinate, fat binders, the ear patch, slimming soaps (aaahahaha), diet magnets, weight loss insoles, exercise pills in a bottle, weight loss in a bottle, (if you're reading some of these thinking, hmmm, haven't tried that one—please call a therapist)." You get the picture. Now you can understand why it is a $50 billion industry. And we are the people making them rich.

Let's start a curvaceous revolution. Flip the coin around. Upset the apple cart. Piss off all those people getting rich off your ignorance and desperation. A desperation that has been fueled by the factors we listed at the beginning of the book. Media, friends, family, society. Let's giggle when the diet industry no longer holds the power—we hold the power. We establish what is acceptable. Curves, butts, laughter, droopy boobs, cellulite, independence, brown hair, crooked teeth, contentment. Let's look up to people like Queen Latifah, Wynona Judd, Oprah Winfrey, Jann Arden, Rita McNeil, Buddha, Santa Claus, Nia Vardalos, Nell Carter, Aretha Franklin, Luisa Tetrazzini (late 19th century opera diva for whom chicken tetrazzini was named), Mama Cass, Tyra Banks, Missy Elliott, your mom, your sister, your friend, your neighbor. Let's jiggle when we run and bounce when we walk. Let's embrace the parts of us that we would like to change and show off the parts of us that we are proud of.

I participate in a program called Bikrams Yoga. Just for a little clarification, Mia and yoga are not two words you would generally find in the same sentence. I'm the type of person that listens to AC/DC, cranked, on the way to yoga, and then cranked on the way home. I fidget when I'm supposed to be still and my mind wanders like a nomad who just won the lottery. But this particular yoga has my name written all over it.

A 40 degree room and 52 tough postures—enough to keep my A.D.D in check. A little digression but one of the things I appreciate about this yoga program are the different shapes and sizes that arrive, half-naked, and ready to sweat. Women who are 30, 40, 50 pounds overweight—wearing as little as possible without pornography music playing in the background. If they are embarrassed or intimidated by the stickish-looking people in the class, they sure don't show it. There is cellulite, crooked boobs, big boobs, huge boobs, no boobs, butt tattoos, short legs, fat arms, thick waists, back fat, and double chins—but who cares? We are all there for one reason—to take care of ourselves. To get fit, to detox, to improve posture and flexibility, to increase strength and stamina and work on mind control. We don't care about who is next to us or what they are wearing. We don't care who can bend more or hold a posture longer. Half the time we don't even notice the other people in the room. If only we could do that when we left the room. Continue to not care what everyone else is wearing or what everyone else looks like and continue to just care about our health—physical and mental. That is what life is all about—not what you look like in your casket but how long it takes you to get there.

Commitment to change.

Commitment, pledge, vow, promise, guarantee, obligation, duty. When you get married you commit yourself to love, honor and cherish your partner. When you are hired for a job you commit to do the best job you can, each and every day. When you are accepted into university you commit to study, learn and work. When you have children you commit to be the best parent that you can be. When you finally decide to engage in a permanent weight loss system you commit to making life-style changes, for life. No more closet eating. No more marathon *Desperate Housewives* on Saturday. No more slipping through

McDonald's drive-thru on your way home from work. No more excuses. No more blaming. No more eating your emotions. No more, just this one time. No more diets. Permanent lifestyle changes equals success.

I listened to one woman tell me how she had been trying for more than 10 years to lose weight and she just kept on getting fatter. Nothing seemed to work. When I asked her what she had tried in the past, she explained the usual stuff such as getting up every morning to walk before the rest of the family got up. Packing her own lunch. No more fancy coffees. No more second helpings. No more late night eating. No more junk food. No more binge drinking. The more she went on, the more confused I got. I began to think that maybe I was wrong and all those things don't work. So I asked her how long she had tried these lifestyle changes for and she said, "Oh, you know, a week here and a week there, but I didn't see any results so I would just give up". Aaahh. Weakly committed. Sort of committed. Would like the results but not the work.

Her exercise program would last about five days or until the weekend arrived. She would last three or four days packing her lunch until she got bored of the choices. She got tired of "depriving" herself of her favorite double-decaf-soymilk-latte with a triple-shot of pumpkin-spice-light-on-the-whip cream but go for it with the chocolate-sauce, coffee. She made excuses as to why she should get to enjoy her fourth glass of wine with dinner and her bag of light popcorn while watching back-to-back episodes of *The Vanity Insanity*. There was absolutely no commitment. There was intention but intention without commitment is just another broken promise. It is another lie tucked away into your subconscious. Another layer of broken promises that the subconscious recognizes as a pattern of failure. Don't wish it—believe it—then, believe in yourself.

Believe in Yourself

Believe in yourself --
in the power you have
to control your own life,
day by day.
Believe in the strength
that you have deep inside,
and your faith will help
show you the way...

Believe in tomorrow
and what it will bring --
let a hopeful heart
carry you through...

For things will work out
if you trust and believe
there's no limit
to what you can do!

Always Believe in You,
Listen to your heart.
Trust your instincts.
Know you CAN.
See your own strengths.
Dream it -- dare it.
Do what you are afraid of.
Keep the faith.
Follow your vision...
Remember ANYTHING is possible
if only you believe.

Unknown author.

Face your F.E.A.R.

Fine **E**at **A**nother **R**ound
Food **E**nds **A**nother **R**age
Forever **E**ating **A**nd **R**unning
Fighting **E**ndlessly **A**fter **R**espect
Free **E**verything **A**bout **R**eality
Forget **E**verything **A**nd **R**un
Fury, **E**vade, **A**ttitude, **R**ise-up
Forbid, **E**liminate, **A**ccept, **R**eact
Forget, **E**nd, **A**ttack, **R**espond
Feel, **E**at, **A**nger, **R**esentment
Fight **E**ach **A**ngry **R**esponse
Find **E**very **A**mbition **R**ealistic
Find **E**verything **A**ll **R**ight

Whatever acronym you wish to spin off F.E.A.R. the outcome is the same—a reluctance to change based on discomfort of the unknown. Will I lose friends if I lose weight? What will happen if I join an exercise class? What am I going to replace my food addiction with? If I admit I have a problem what are people going to think about me? Will people think I am weak? Will people laugh at me? What will I have in common with my friends? What if I fail again? The questions go on and on until your fear overcomes your desire for change. When this happens your dreams get swept away—again. If you don't overcome the fear that holds you back, you will never be able to achieve your goals. Unlike thousands of years ago when fear was necessary for survival, today most of our fears are created in our minds.

We perceive failing before we even start, therefore it is safer to not start. Sadly, if we let fear rule our life we become a victim of it. Then we quit living and start just surviving.

What is the worst thing that could happen? You don't start. Everything else is a perceived fear. Sure it is going to be uncomfortable but will it be more uncomfortable than how you feel now? Are you going to be hungry? Probably, but that will go away. Are you going to feel deprived? Possibly, if you try to go cold turkey. Are you going to have days where you fall? Likely, but it doesn't really matter as long as you get back up. Are you going to look at your favorite tub of ice-cream and long to eat it all? Yup, but the results are going to make you strong. Are you going to lose some of your food-addicted cronies? If you do, were they really friends? Are people going to be watching and waiting for you to fail? Depends on what type of people you choose to surround yourself with. And on and on and on.

Fear holds back so many women from achieving their weight loss goals and from letting go of their food addictions. For some women, it is their best friend. Always around through boredom, stress, sadness, loneliness, failure, jealousy. Instead of letting fear hold you back from your successes in life, why not just take it on the trip. Pack it up and stick it in your back pocket. If you need it it's there and if you don't, forget about it. Eventually, you will make peace with your fear and learn to use it to your advantage and not your disadvantage.

Initially, I had a huge fear of writing this book. I had absolutely no idea what the hell I was doing. I didn't know how to write a book. I didn't know how to research for a book. I am not a writer. I am not a therapist. I was afraid of not being able to do it. I was afraid of not being able to find women to participate in the project. I was afraid of not working. I was afraid of getting a big, fat writer's butt. I would wake up in the middle of the night wondering what I had gotten myself into. Could I have picked a more difficult topic? Who is going to buy this book? Who is going to publish the book? Who will want to sell this book? Who will listen to what I have to say? Who is going to take me seriously?' Every time one of those thoughts would enter my mind, I would shut it off because I was afraid of the answer. Eventually, I just decided what is the worst that could happen? I meet a bunch of interesting women. I get to research a burning question that I have had for years. I get to learn. I get to expand my knowledge in many new areas. I get to experience something completely different and exciting.

Well, I am six months into the project and I no longer worry about any of those things. I have learned so much about people, writing, publishing, marketing, formatting, myself and of course, dieting. I know that something will come of this project —what, remains to be seen. I have received tremendous support and encouragement from the community. Not only do I not worry about the success of the book anymore, but I am already thinking about the next book. Not because I think this one will be such a resounding success but because I have never enjoyed anything so much in my life as writing and researching. I set my own hours. I get as much exercise as I like. I get to go to every one of our sons activities. I get to be there for him before, during and after school. I make sure there is always plenty of good home cooking in the house. The house is always clean and the laundry is always done. I get to have lunch with friends. I get to read and read and read. I get to have massages. I get to go for long bike rides in the middle of the day. Had I listened to my fears, I never would have embarked on this journey.

We all have hopes and we all have dreams. Taking the uncomfortable and scary steps necessary to achieve them is what sets the successful apart from the ordinary. Don't be afraid to hope and to dream and if one of your hopes and one of your dreams is to change the way you look and the way you feel,

take the appropriate steps. No more quick fixes. No more gimmicks. No more, *just this once*. No more diets. No more, *I'll
start tomorrow*. No more, *I don't have the time or the money*.
No more excuses.

The four E's to successful weight management.

Education
Eat responsibly
Exercise daily
Enjoy life!

12
WISDOM

From every experience in life comes knowledge. Choosing to learn from the experience, positive or negative, is up to us. Part of the Buddhist belief is the philosophy called *The Eight Winds*. Gain and loss, praise and ridicule, credit and blame and suffering and joy. These *Eight Winds* struggle inside us constantly. If we don't learn to recognize these feelings then they have the opportunity to control us instead of us controlling them.

Having the freedom to make choices is one of the many gifts we have as Canadians. Our choices have the opportunity to imprison us or to set us free. It is called the freedom of choice or free will. How we choose to live our lives, how we choose to treat others and how we choose to treat ourselves is ultimately our choice and our choice alone.

As we get older, generally speaking, we become wiser. We become calmer, more centered and more content. As we head toward menopause or are in the midst of menopause we b e g i n the journey home. Home to a place we once occupied before puberty. A place where we are once again free to become the centre of our own lives. A place where we are once again confident, self-directed, self-motivated, and full of energy. Free to look as we please and to dress the way we like—a way that is no longer determined by our friends, our peers or the media. We have picked up a lot of luggage along this journey, some pieces we have kept, some we have hauled to the dump. Many times one of these pieces of luggage is full of food issues, dysfunctional eating, eating disorders and weight issues. Sometimes we carry it along our journey to the end, other times we take it to the intellectual dump and leave it for the vultures.

Food and eating disorders can be very addictive. People eat or drink or do drugs or have dangerous sex so they don't have to feel. Whatever the drug of choice is, people do it so they don't have to feel emotions that are overwhelming such as fear, anger, loneliness, boredom, sadness or anxiety. They eat to medicate emotional pain. If they felt harmony, contentment or peace, they wouldn't require a mood altering "drug" in order to find peace.

Eating disorders are a very interesting irony. They are about ultimate control when everything else in life is out of control. But someone caught in the vise of an eating disorder or weight loss struggle surrenders control *to* the obsession. It is not them that is in control but the struggle which ultimately controls them. This holds true for chronic dieters.

In time, I hope women get to the root of why they eat or don't eat or overeat. In order to conquer their dysfunctional food habits they are going to have to identify what makes them feel they have to medicate with food. If they are lonely, they need to join a class or volunteer or reach out to friends, not eat the loneliness. If they are overworked and overtired, they need to take some time to rest, not eat the fatigue. If they are anxious, they need to identify the source of their anxiety and learn from it, not eat the anxiety. If they are angry, they need to remove themselves from the situation that makes them angry, not eat the anger. Sounds easy—maybe sometimes it is.

Learning to stop and think; think to recognize; recognize to accept; accept to learn, will eventually guide us down the road to acceptance. Acceptance of others and acceptance of ourselves. Realizing that our body is a gift, regardless of the shape. *It* is what makes babies. *It* is what runs marathons. *It* is what teaches. *It* is what walks. *It* is what makes love. *It* is what goes on vacation. *It* is what drives the kids to school. Without *it* there is no walking, teaching, making love, having babies, experiencing life. Acceptance of oneself is not a destination or a place to aspire to, it is a journey. A journey of discovery, consciousness, intention, change and hope.

My dear friend brilliantly answered the question, 'Can you recall a single moment in time when someone said something or did something that changed the way you thought about your body?' like this: "No, I have a mirror. I don't need anyone to tell me my areas of improvement, and I don't really give a shit what they think anyway. That is why they invented clothes!" She is the same wise person when I asked if being thin equaled happiness and success she said, "No, being happy equals success".

Wise people have learned to *live* life and not just *do* life. Whether you are the type of person that believes in reincarnation or not, until I am introduced to Elvis Presley or Lady Diana, in the flesh, I believe we have one life to live, in this body, and we better enjoy every single moment of every single hour of every single day because in the blink of an eye, it is over. Our spirit and our soul may live on but it needs a body in order to live so we better learn to love the one we have because it is the only one we've got.

So what if you are 20 pounds overweight and your left boob is bigger than your right, your hair is curly instead of straight and you're two inches shorter than your sister. So what. So what. So what. Who are you inside? I challenge you to sit down and write a positive statement about yourself. A statement about your spirit. Your true-self, not your *earth suit* as one little Grade 5 student called it. Your *earth suit* is like the husk on a cob of corn, it doesn't say anything about the sweetness inside. Are you kind, are you compassionate, are you loving, are you smart, are you witty? What makes you who you are? Now focus on that statement and learn to start living life through your description of your spirit not your earth suit.

The path to healing starts with learning to love yourself. I know you're thinking, "Yeah, yeah, enough already, I've heard it a hundred times". It is time to start listening. Loving yourself doesn't mean you have to make love to yourself! It doesn't mean you have to stand in front of the mirror, naked, singing your praises every day. It doesn't mean telling your friends what a glorious, wonderful human being you are. It doesn't mean taking out a billboard asking people to send you money for a new home because you are so fabulous your head doesn't fit inside your current home anymore. It means recognize and admit that you have some fabulous qualities. Focus on those qualities and let them surface. Start spending your day looking at ways to utilize your great attributes rather than wondering how you're going to make your right boob bigger. If more people in the world recognized and nurtured their spirit, the world would all of a sudden become a better place. Instead, it is a *me* society. Everything is about what benefits *me*.

"It's ironic that at 20 we have it all. A cute figure, great hair, great skin, no responsibilities, and a spunky metabolism but we are never content. Then at 40 or 50, we don't have any of the things we had at 20, but we have contentment."
Interview client #50

"You should love yourself. If you don't you will always wish you were someone else."   **Interview client #74**

"Am I happy with myself—much more than I was yesterday or the day before and a little less than I will be tomorrow."
Interview client #46

"I love myself in many ways, I just hate the package I came in."
Interview client #60

"I think it is possible to love yourself you just have to start by accepting the stuff you can't change."
Interview client #50

"If you can't love yourself where you are at then you'll never be able to love yourself."   **Interview client #47**

"Always remember that you are someone's goal weight."
Interview client #46

"I try to keep loving myself by facing each day as I get older. I try to be the best I can be without getting down on myself because there is another wrinkle or my thighs aren't as tight as they used to be."   **Interview client #36**

Serenity, courage, wisdom.

The serenity prayer. *God grant me the serenity to accept the things I cannot change*, (height, genetics, set-point), *courage to change the things I can*, (exercise, nutrition, dieting), *wisdom to know the difference*, (thinness does not equal happiness and fatness does not equal unhappiness).

Many women I spoke with made comments such as, "You have no idea what it is like to be fat", "People like you just don't understand", "Try living in my shoes", "You are the type of person that everyone wants to look like". Whenever these comments were made, I would say, "You're right, I don't know what it is like", "I have never walked in your shoes", "Maybe I don't understand and perhaps some people would like to be my height and weight," but I also think, what does that have to do with life? What does it truly have to do with life? You could say, "Everything. If I just wasn't fat or if I was just thinner, everything in life would be better." So then, if that is what you think, then do something about it. I don't mean that in a way that is meant to be flippant or simplistic but in order to truly change that which holds you back you are going to have to get scared and uncomfortable. The author, Denis Waitley, says, "A dream is your creative vision for your life in the future. You must break out of your current comfort zone and become comfortable with the unfamiliar and the unknown."

The women I spoke with that were no longer on the diet journey learned that facing their fear was the first step to eliminating their fear. The fear of failing. The fear of never being skinny. The fear of not being loved. The fear of not being pretty enough. The fear of not being successful. The fear of changing. Once they admitted the fear, they took the first step toward a new life. The same as an alcoholic admitting they are an alcoholic. The first step is admitting there is a problem.

Keep in mind we have established that being overweight is not necessarily a problem but rather, thinking that being skinny, is the key to happiness. Letting the scale dictate your daily moods is a problem; getting rid of the scale is facing your fear. Secretly hiding food and eating it when no one is around is a problem; telling your loved ones is facing your fear. Hating your body is a problem; changing that attitude is facing your fear. Not exercising is a problem; joining a fitness class is facing your fear. Break it down into manageable steps because no task is impossible if you break it down into small enough steps.

Clarity is a gift.

So many women muddle through life in a haze of tasks never stopping long enough to stand up and poke their heads through the miasma of life in order to see the clarity above the clouds. Every wise person I have ever met has a sense of calm or serenity about them. It doesn't matter how chaotic the world around them appears, they seem to create an aura of calm. I believe this is clarity. They witness life as a whole scene, in great detail. It is like a person knowing they are about to be involved in a car crash and they say everything just seemed to move in slow motion. I believe part of the demise of the female self-esteem is the haze of life that has been deposited upon our laps. Granted, we have taken on that role and must be accountable. At the same time, we never asked for it all. Mother, wife, maid, chauffeur, cook, counselor, gardener, fit, beautiful, sexy, charming, funny, loving, caring, supportive, nurturing, munch, munch, munch. Husband, on the other hand. Work. If we could just get a bit of clarity about our life, our perspective would change. If our perspective changed, our priorities would change. If our priorities changed, we would start taking care of ourselves first, so that we had the mental health and energy to take care of everyone and everything else in our lives.

> *How we choose to live our life*
> *and how we choose to treat our body*
> *is our choice and our choice only.*

"I am very aware that it is about choice but I just want what other people so freely choose without suffering the consequences."   **Interview client #60**

"I believe that we only have one body and one life and we don't need to abuse it to enjoy life. We need to care about ourselves as much as we care about others."
Interview client #41

"I feel that we can decide what we want to do or how we want to look. Nobody makes us a certain way or makes those decisions but us. There is no use blaming anyone for your decisions."   **Interview client #40**

"We need to learn to accept that as we age our body changes and that we won't be who we were when we were younger—my outlook has changed to one of acceptance."
Interview client #40

> *Wisdom is knowing where to go from here.*

'*Ignorance is Bliss*', ends here. As the famous English writer, Aldous Huxley once said, "Facts do not cease to exist because they are ignored".

Wisdom comes from experience and from the knowledge that is acquired through experience. Each and every diet or failed attempt at weight loss is an experience. It has provided you with knowledge that you may or may not realize is catalogued under life experiences. What you choose to do with those life experiences, with the knowledge and with the facts that you have now acquired will determine where you will be one month, six months or one year from now. I invite you to use the tools you possess in your intellectual handbag to establish or re-establish appropriate life changes that will deliver you to the personal vision you have for your future.

13
THE PERFECT ME

Writing this book has taught me that being content with who you are and what you look like has to begin inside of you. It has taught me that the journey to contentment is a long, difficult and painful trip but the destination is worth the struggle. The destination is one of dignity and understanding. I would like to invite you to be who you are with dignity and with pride. Be short with dignity. Be overweight with dignity. Be boobless with dignity. Be fat with dignity. Be single with dignity. Be a woman with dignity. Without dignity and without pride the journey to contentment will never end and there will never be a "perfect you". You will never enjoy life through your own eyes if you spend your whole life trying to be someone other than who you are. Start living today. Start by recognizing that you are perfect just the way you are. Best selling author, Robert Collier said, "Success is the sum of small efforts, repeated day in and day out".

"The illusion of perfect would be as follows: waking up in the morning without fear or anxiety about all of the unknowns that the day will hold. To not question or worry about all of the things that I am supposed to know. To be comfortable with allowing myself to live my life as I choose as opposed to the way others think I should live. I would be fit, without the worry of obsession sneaking back into my life, and I would be happy with myself. I would be less afraid of losing control because of a developed stronger sense of trust in myself."
Interview client #5

"I like my mind and even though it's not a perfect body, I still like my body."   **Interview client #71**

Sometimes weight loss can surprise us. We think if we could just lose 30 pounds we would be happy. When we finally reach our goal, we find we are no happier than we were when we were 30 pounds heavier. Just because we change the outside of us doesn't mean we have changed the inside of us and the inside is where the change must begin. Internal changes versus external appearance. Just because you are beautiful on the outside does not mean you are beautiful on the inside. The old saying "You can't judge a book by its cover," is tired and simple, but true.

Our *earth suit* is what we are born with and we live in. It is our brown hair, our green eyes, our short legs, our cowlick and birthmark, it is our height and our weight and it is our skin color. It has nothing to do with who we truly are. Who we truly are comes from our hearts and our souls, the very part of us that gets destroyed trying so desperately to change our *earth suit*. Simply—our *earth suit* is what holds our spirit.

Asking women what the *perfect me* meant to them was as

interesting as it was diverse. If the woman being interviewed was older and had more life experiences, her answer tended to reflect more about her spirituality. If the woman was still struggling with her desperate journey, her answer tended to be more about size, shape and weight. If the woman was raised in a functional, healthy environment, her answer tended to be more about health and fitness.

The *perfect me* question is as profound and confusing as puberty. Take a look at the following words and determine which ones reflect who you think you are and which ones reflect who you would like to be and observe how far apart or how close together those character traits are.

Loving, caring, happy, arrogant, witty, intelligent, warm-hearted, nurturing, self-centered, vain, content, whole, motivated, determined, kind, reliable, organized, healthy, fit, moral, ethical, bright, shy, extroverted, bubbly, funny, vivacious, attentive, compassionate, sympathetic, forthright, approachable, hospitable, self-serving, giving, courageous, brave, angry, gregarious, a leader, successful, confused, a listener, a follower, unassuming, bitter, reserved, uptight, spiritual, wise, cooperative, indulgent, goal-oriented, confident, jealous, cunning, driven, secure, independent, competent, a perfectionist, honest, true, complete.

Those character traits that you have define your soul and have nothing to do with your *earth suit*. Those character traits that you wish to have, describe the *perfect you*. How can we go about utilizing the character traits were born with, in order to help us develop the character traits we wish to possess? The *perfect me* is who we are when we think no one else is looking.

"The perfect me is imperfect."   **Interview client #12**

We are all perfectly imperfect human beings.

"The perfect me is exactly who I am at 220 pounds but with the ability to say 'no' without feeling guilty."
Interview client #24

"A fit 150 pounds who no longer snores!"
Interview client #51

"The perfect me is less wiggly and jello-y!"
Interview client #46

"The perfect me is me. I am so blessed. I accept my shortcomings and embrace my strengths." **Interview client #39**

"The perfect me would be a bit taller and my right elbow would be as nice as my left elbow."
Student

"The perfect me talks a little less!" **Interview client #30**

"The perfect me would be at peace with my obsession over body image."
Interview client #13

"I think I am the perfect me, minus the nail biting!"
Student

"The perfect me is content being alone!"
Interview client #22

"The perfect me is proud and happy on the inside."
Interview client #19

"The perfect me would be five foot four with straight toes."
Student

"Is it possible to love yourself? Yes, if you can accept the ways you disappoint yourself." **Interview client #30**

"The perfect me is freckle-free, eyes farther apart, bigger breasts and narrower hips, more positive and patient with my-self and my family." **Interview client #20**

"When I was 25 years old and had no fat rolls hanging over my bra and out over my underwear." **Interview client #41**

"The perfect me is 10 pounds lighter than what I am but I know that is dangerous given my past relationship with food and dieting." **Interview client #38**

"One hundred ten pounds or less." **Interview client #44**

"The perfect me is calmer, at peace, mentally quiet and non-judgmental." **Interview client #64**

"The perfect me has firmer skin on my face, no age spots, firmer breasts, no saggy stretch marks or ugly belly button, no hemorrhoids, no herpes, no depression—happy, healthy, confi-dent, motivated with lots of friends. When I can start growing old gracefully and when I don't need compliments." **Interview client #62**

"The perfect me is fit, slender, blemish free, stretch mark-free and cottage cheese-free." **Interview client #42**

"The perfect me has no belly fat but is strong looking, not skinny." **Interview client #40**

"Omm—tight thighs, a butt you can bounce a quarter off and a healthy body." **Interview client #36**

Believe in who you are.

Success starts by believing in yourself. You'll notice in the last chapter of this book many of the women thanked themselves for their weight loss and lifestyle successes. They knew the only way they were going to truly succeed at their weight loss endeavors was by believing they could do it. Even if everyone else around them told them they couldn't or wouldn't, they shut out the naysayers and listened to their inside voice.

Our kids, our husbands, our employers, our pets, our neighbors, our churches and our volunteer organizations believe in us, but often we don't believe in ourselves. If you tell yourself over and over and over that you will never lose weight, that this diet won't work, that you can't stick to an exercise program, that you can't resist the Wagon Wheels rolling around in the cupboard, your subconscious will begin to recognize that thought pattern and determine the outcome. You start a new diet knowing you won't stick to it. You start a new exercise program and you know you won't commit to it. You vow to quit closet eating while you're thinking about those damn Wagon Wheels. If you don't believe you can do it, then you can't. If you believe you can do it, then you will.

Start your new approach to weight loss by giving yourself the credit you deserve. Don't look for outside affirmation, tell yourself you can and you will change those old thought patterns from *I can't*, to *I will*. Even if no one else believes you can do it, believe in yourself and know you will.

"If you can't love yourself where you are at, then you'll never be able to love yourself. If you can take your eyes off of yourself for just a minute, you'll see life isn't that bad."

Interview client #47

Self-love/self-worth/self-esteem?

Weight and self-image are not the same thing. They are not interchangeable. Being too thin or being too large does not determine our self-worth, *we* determine our self-worth. Food and weight and body image do not define who we are, just like our spouse, the car we drive and our job do not define who we are. What lives inside of us defines who we are. Our self-worth is the quality or qualities we are born with that make us worthwhile. Our strengths and our value as human beings. Everyone is born with self-worth but many lose it along life's complicated journey. When we lose sight of our self-worth our self-esteem dwindles and when our self-esteem dwindles it is impossible to love ourselves. If we can't love ourselves, we can't truly love others.

"It's hard to love yourself, if you haven't been loved."
Interview client #39

I interviewed a 35-year-old woman who had a psychology degree and worked in the Human Resource Department of a large resort. She was intelligent, beautiful, funny, and yes, overweight and she knew all of these things were true. When I asked her questions such as, 'Explain what self-worth means to you or does being skinny mean happiness and success?' I was constantly surprised by her answers. She truly believed that if she were skinny, her life would be perfect. She would be a better mother, a better wife, a better boss. People would view her differently, they would respect her more and she would be more successful. Her husband would be more attracted to her, (although he already was) and she would be able to love herself. Her father would tell her how proud he was of her and that gnawing feeling would go away. When I asked her if she truly believed in her heart, that losing weight would make all of those things better, she was adamant that it would. She is the same person who answered, 'If I were skinny', to the question, 'Could you love yourself?'

"Self-worth is how and what makes you, you. It is the identification in all of us. My self-worth is a life long process of millions of pieces that cling together and float apart. Sometimes the pieces fit like a puzzle and are complete—other times the pieces don't fit and must be moved around to make self-worth complete. It is a very fragile state."

Interview client #40

"Self-worth is nothing but a state of mind. It can give charm to one's personality or it can destroy the heart. Poor self-worth discourages friendships and invites disaster, leading us to misery. Healthy self-worth shapes one's chances of achievement in any situation. It allows love to happen and opens the heart, willpower and perseverance."

Interview client #55

"Self-worth is valuing yourself enough as a person, that you are comfortable with your decisions, making you a leader and not a follower."   **Interview client #53**

"Self-worth is how valuable I am to the world."

Interview client #46

"To have dignity and pride in yourself and your actions."

Student

"How you look at yourself in the mirror."   **Student**

"Self-worth, like integrity, is who you are when no one is looking."   **Student**

"How you feel about yourself and how much you value and like yourself."   **Student**

"Self-worth is to value who you are in the present."   **Student**

"Self-worth, to me, would have to be the contribution that I have to society and those around me."   **Student**

"If you are content."   **Student**

"Knowing that you are important and have a purpose in life."   **Student**

"I am a unique and talented individual with an open mind and occasionally an enlightened world view and to me that is self-worth."   **Student**

"Knowing my boundaries."   **Student**

"Self-worth is your price tag, relative to how you view the worth of others. How much you feel you contribute to this world, how much you will be missed when you are gone, and how important it is that you are here."
                                      Interview client #42

"In my eyes I guess I see self-worth as something that just sets you free. If you place a high value on yourself, you can do any-thing, if you place a low value on yourself, it leads to self-punishing cycles of disorders."   **Interview client #13**

"Having pride, respect and confidence in myself, as much as possible."   **Interview client #41**

"Being proud of who you are."   **Interview client #36**

"Self-worth is how a person feels about themselves. When they take the good with the bad and tally it up, hopefully the good outweighs the bad."   **Interview client #30**

"To me self-worth is putting yourself first and not compromising your beliefs or your morals—loving yourself and never putting yourself down."   **Interview client #73**

What affects your self-worth?

Self-loathing and negative self-talk were the two biggest factors in how women felt about themselves. They would play negative self-talk tapes over and over in their heads until they began to believe what they were thinking. Little things, such as someone not saying hello could become, 'She hates me because of the way I look', where in fact, she just didn't see you. Telling yourself that your husband doesn't want to have sex with you because you are so disgusting, could be that you are the one giving off the vibes that you don't want to be touched because you are so uncomfortable with your body. Telling yourself that you couldn't possibly join a gym because everyone would stare at your fat body, keeps you from getting fit. Telling yourself over and over that your life will be better once you lose the weight, causes you to believe that your life isn't okay the way it is. We have to learn to pop those tapes out and replace them with a comedy tape or an Oprah Winfrey tape or a, *Damn, I Look Fine* tape. It's tough but you can do it.

Putting everyone else before oneself was a huge factor in diminished self-worth and self-esteem. This was so typical of women with children. I believe we are not only taught that everyone and everything comes first—husband, children, job, laundry, toilets, dishes, groceries, errands, soccer practice, music lessons, gymnastics, dance, the cat, the dog, the horse, the friggin' neighbor's kids and animals, but that we inherently feel that way as women. I found that concept very easy to get over, right from the start, and I don't think that makes me selfish, I think it makes me wise. I figured out right away if I didn't keep exercise as a priority no one was going to want to be around me! Even when our son was born, minus 30 degrees in Saskatoon in the middle of December, I was bundled up with him inside of a snuggly inside of my coat, getting out for my walk. I rented a Stairmaster for the living room and stepped my little buns off. I was lucky because my job was always in the fitness industry but there were many days when the last thing I wanted to do was exercise because I just wanted to get away from fitness. It was never an option. I learned that exercising was for me and it was about me, no one else. I didn't care if I was faster, stronger, fitter, leaner, more flexible than another person or another athlete. That was not the point. The point was to take the time for me and to love what I was doing at that time. It ultimately made me a happier, calmer, healthier person with more energy, clarity and ambition. Women have to learn to take time for themselves, it is essential. It could be 10 minutes or a half hour. It might be a bath, a walk, lunch with friends, the gym, a television show or meditation. It doesn't really matter what, it just matters that we do. When we take time for ourselves, we learn things about ourselves and sometimes, that is the fear we need to face.

Making mistakes. Don't be afraid to make them. No one is perfect—not even Oprah! Learn from your mistakes, it is one of the greatest lessons in life. Learn from all the times you dieted and it didn't work. Learn that not exercising makes you unhealthy and unfit. Learn that not eating breakfast slows down your metabolism. Mistakes are one of the few free lessons in life (the outcome might not be but the mistake itself is). You don't have to buy a book, take a course or go to a special school. You can pretty much be guaranteed that mistakes will just happily present themselves in your life, forever, and what you do with those mistakes determines whether you get an A in that lesson or an F. For most of my early adulthood I would say I got Es in most of my life mistake lessons, but I believe I've graduated to the 'effort honor roll' and am getting a few Bs and the odd A! I've learned that it's okay to be perfectly imperfect.

Finally, quit trying to be someone or something you are not. When I asked the young girls in Grades 4 through 6 who they would most like to be like or look like, the majority of them said themselves, with the exception of one little girl who said she wanted to look just like her horse. To varying degrees, we as human beings, spend a good portion of our lives wanting what we don't have and wishing we were someone we are not. If we could only harness all that energy and put it into turning off those negative self-talk tapes, hop on our bikes, and not be afraid to accidentally put our helmet on backwards, we would be on our way to improving our self-worth.

"I have wasted so much brain space and time focusing on my weight and my body image." **Interview client #44**

If being "skinny" is what motivates you then put it into perspective. Find balance in your life while working toward your "skinny" goal. Nurture your mind and your spirit and your body will change, along with the way you perceive your body. Don't be afraid to admit that being "skinny" or losing weight is important to you but don't let it control your life any longer. Use your goal of weight loss as your motivator. Focus on moving toward your goal. Enjoy the process. Look forward to the destination. Learn from the set-backs.

From this point forward, do not allow your body, your size or your weight define who you are. Do not let those perceptions determine your self-worth. Become a better you and enjoy traveling through life in this suit.

14

MOTIVATORS

A motivator is someone who moves another into action. Motivation is the psychological feature that arouses us into action, toward a desired goal. Motivation and motivators are ongoing and essential to success. Author and motivational speaker Zig Ziglar once said, "People often say that motivation doesn't last. Well, neither does bathing—that's why we recommend it daily." Weight loss and healthy self-esteem require a tremendous amount of motivation on a daily basis, from morning until night. What motivates us to move toward our goal is very different from person to person, even if the goal is the same. If your goal is to lose weight, the reason behind that goal has to be greater than that which keeps you at this weight, such as health issues, relationship issues, self- esteem, a dress size, a wedding. You will have to be very motivated to be uncomfortable, to give things up, and to change.

What motivates you? Is it your children, your health, your marriage, your job, your desires, your happiness? Is it enough motivation to move you to change? Is it enough motivation to move you to be very uncomfortable? If not, you will have to find what does. It may be a person, it may be the goal or the desire itself. Regardless, something motivates us all. For me, it is my overall quality of life that motivates me. The great thing about my motivation is that I will never get there. As life continues to get better, I keep raising the bar. The more fit I get, the more fit I want to be. The more difficult a challenge becomes, the more difficult I want the next challenge to be. The more traveling I do, the more traveling I want to do. Someone who tells me I can't do something, motivates me to make sure I can. The happier I am, the happier I want to be. The more goals I achieve, the more goals I set.

Motivation comes from within. It can be encouraged, promoted and enthused but it can't be bought, ordered, picked up or baked. It starts by believing in you.

Replacing "I can't" with "I can".

Part of our *can't* response is based on previous experiences. If you tried 20 times in the past to stick to a gym program and couldn't but you sign up for another two year contract, somewhere in the back of your mind, you know you won't stick to it, based on previous experiences. It's the same with dieting. Most women know, in the back of their mind, what is the expected outcome based on so many failed attempts. You can have all the motivation and education you want, but unless you change the way you think, the outcome will be the same. Instead of thinking *I can't and won't ever lose weight*, start saying *I can and I will*. You may not know how, but eventually your brain will to start to believe you can and take over some of the confusion for you. I guarantee that hidden away in your subconscious, your brain knows about eating breakfast, staying away from high-sugar and processed foods, that exercise is good for you, that eating at night isn't and that diets don't work. If you started to say, 'I *can* stay away from food at night, I *can* make time to exercise, I *can* avoid McDonald's and I *will* eat breakfast,' it will eventually become a new message in your conscious brain. Start to see yourself the way you want to look and the way you want your life to be and eventually your brain will recognize that as the new response and will move you towards your goal rather than towards another failed attempt. I worked with so many women throughout my fitness career that told me they couldn't. They couldn't lift that, they couldn't run an 8 km run, they couldn't lose weight, they couldn't make it through a spin class, they couldn't fix their back, they couldn't, couldn't, couldn't. I didn't just tell them they could, I proved to them they could. It always amazed me that they couldn't see their potential but a stranger could.

If my husband and I believed every time the bank said we couldn't make a go of a fitness centre, we never would have opened Fitness Excellence, one of the most successful facilities on Vancouver Island. We went to every bank and were rejected every time. Eventually we started over again but brought reinforcements with us. People that supported and believed in the project. Finally we found a bank that agreed.

If someone tells me I can't—I do! As I am writing this book, I have no idea how I am going to get it published. I probably have a better chance of winning the lottery than finding a publishing company to publish this book but the challenge makes me giggle. I'll be persistent to a fault. I'll be like an annoying, little rat dog that never shuts up. I'll send a letter to every reputable publishing company and if they all decline, I'll start over with a different letter. The challenge motivates me. You have to start by replacing *I can't*, with *I will*.

I felt it would be a gift to those people who motivated the women I spoke with, to recognize them in their own chapter, after all, many of these women said they couldn't have done it without them. They deserve recognition today and every day for helping to make another human being's quality of life, better. When you are scanning this list to see if your name is on it, take a look at how many women thanked themselves for their success. Those women replaced *I can't* with *I can* and they believed in themselves.

- Myself—for not giving in and letting this take over my entire life. Never giving up.
- My daughter Olivia (14 months old).
- My mother.
- David Summers.
- Shirley Wade-Linton.
- Maggie St. Aubrey.
- Esther Crane.
- God.
- Friends.
- Cindy.
- Oprah.
- My husband.
- Mia.
- My husband.
- Myself and all my counselors along the way.
- Herself.
- My friends. I have been blessed with amazing friends.
- My own inner resources.
- Over-Eater's Anonymous.
- My children for putting up with me.
- Mom, she hasn't done something in particular, she was just always there.
- My ex-boyfriend.

- Myself.
- Myself, but I did it for my parents.
- I would like to thank all the people who have hung in there with me. Who have tried to love me when I have been unlovable. Those that taught me how to love others and myself. People at the gym who have encouraged me.
- My mother.
- I could thank a lot of people for a lot of different reasons but most of all I thank me. For not giving up on myself and having the confidence to keep going because I made me what I am today.
- All of those people and friends who had to put up with me saying I'm fat. The folks at the gym who were inspiring.
- Myself for having the strength to persevere. Anyone who inspires me to try harder when I want to give up.
- My family, especially my supportive husband.
- Myself and my ex-husband. He secretly arranged a lunch with a recovered anorectic, to help me on the road to recovery.
- Myself. I always am looking for new ways to learn and to feel good from my experiences.
- My husband who has always been my closest friend and my biggest supporter.
- My parents for loving me for me. My friends for supporting me and my fiancé for helping me get through stressful situations and for making me feel good about myself.
- My husband for thinking I am the most beautiful girl in the world.
- Myself, because there is nothing I won't do that I want to do.
- My clients as I have no family or significant other.
- My sisters for always supporting and encouraging me.
- My husband and myself.
- The group at TOPS.

- My co-workers because most of them are older women who have more life experience and keep me thinking positive about myself.
- My mom and dad.
- Myself.
- You, for getting me to face myself and learn to try and accept myself.
- My good friend who lost 155 pounds and showed me the same path.
- My husband for never ever saying anything about my weight or my body and loving me unconditionally.
- Fitness Excellence and all its wonderful trainers for help and guidance over the years.
- My husband.
- God.
- Everyone I have met that has touched me both positively and negatively, as we learn from both.
- My best friend.
- My husband.
- My best friend.
- My friend, she is so helpful.
- My sisters.
- Myself.
- My parents for giving me the necessary values to survive.
- My son—he is my everything.
- God.
- My yoga instructor.
- My sisters.
- My priest.
- My run group.
- My walking partner.
- Myself.
- Absolutely myself.
- My best friend.

Who motivate me?

My family motivates me. My friends motivate me. My challenges motivate me. Life motivates me. A beautiful, sunny day motivates me. A miserable day motivates me. Exercise motivates me. My son motivates me. But mostly I motivate me.

Two years ago, in 2004, our son, who was 12 at the time, was in a ridiculous motorbike accident that left him with two less fingers and a badly injured ring finger. It was the first day of Christmas holidays. I cried and cried because I couldn't believe something so slow and so innocent could produce such a horrible outcome. After his first of three surgeries, he woke up and I broke the news to him. He was quiet for a moment and then he asked me how much of his fingers were gone and I told him. All he said was, "It is a good thing I didn't lose more of them." One week later, the remainder of one of the fingers, which was badly infected, had to be completely removed. Throughout his ordeal he never cried, he never complained, he smiled and laughed. He opened his Christmas presents with one hand and laughed when he got a hockey stick and a new pair of riding gloves. But I kept on crying because the accident left me so traumatized. One day, shortly after his second surgery he said to me, "Mom, why are you crying?" and I told him it was because I was so sad that he had lost his fingers. He said to me, "Well I'm not sad, so stop crying." He never missed a day of school, and he went right back to playing in the local recreational basketball league one month after his accident. He played for the next three months with one hand and a special cast on his injured hand. He was adamant there was to be no special treatment. He approached his physical therapy sessions with enthusiasm and laughter. He made me realize how much life is about attitude.

Thank you for the opportunity of a lifetime.

I would like to leave you with "Thank you"! Thank you for allowing me the opportunity to learn from your struggles, your experiences and your courage. Thank you for helping me to understand why women feel the way they do about body image, food and weight. Thank you for giving me a glimpse into your lives.

It is my goal and my intention to help women realize how important they are to their families, their communities, their countries and to the world and their importance has nothing to do with their size. Women have the power to affect the greatest change because their motivation comes from love and from peace, not from war. It does not matter how small the town is that you live in or how much you weigh, you make a difference in people's lives and you are making a difference in this world.

I believe women have the ability to be free of this demon called body image and the burden called weight loss. I believe the state of self-absorption that the media has created is going to change. I believe that people like Oprah Winfrey, Ellen DeGeneres, Mother Teresa, Dana Reeve, Lady Diana, Mya Angelou and Hilary Clinton are arousing us out of a victimized state and are fanning the embers of change. Don't ever think you're too small or you can't—if you do, then you are and you won't.

It is with overwhelming gratitude that I wish every woman that reads this book the very best of luck on their journey to personal freedom.

To contact me with your story or for information on other projects I have implemented or am in the process of developing go to www.miasbook.com. I am available for public speaking engagements, seminars and courses. Please feel free to contact me through my website.

Mia Sutherland

ISBN 142511725-2